I Chose Leukemia

And the 49 Truths that Healed Me

Sarah Stevenson

I Chose Leukemia
And The 49 Truths That Healed Me

Sarah Stevenson

© Sarah Stevenson 2025

Zen Barn Publishing, LLC

Sarah Stevenson
Point Pleasant, NJ

ISBN: 979-8-9860235-7-1

www.mindfuleducationalservices.com

Forward

It is day one of my 49-day stay in isolation at Jersey Shore Medical Center in Neptune, NJ. I'm alone. There will be a lot of "alone" time in the days following, and I haven't yet experienced what this might feel like around day 32. I'm here. It's quiet, and I await my first breakfast tray. I'm strangely excited about breakfast in bed. When was the last time I had breakfast in bed in the past twenty years? This prompted me to pick up the hospital menu at my bedside to see what the offerings for lunch and dinner would be. I decided to make my selections closer to the meal times because it's something to look forward to.

Breakfast arrives. Scrambled eggs that looked like they should, but carried a synthetic taste. It's like everything else here. Little Smuckers strawberry packets are stacked neatly alongside the half-buttered white toast. There was a time when I would never dream of allowing myself to eat white bread, butter, and jelly in the same bite. This is the former eating disorder brain at its finest. Always calculate, make judgments, and give you warnings with every food encounter you come across. Does this seem far-fetched and exaggerated? It's not. It's trauma-informed taste buds.

I eat my breakfast slowly and look out the large picture window that will become a boring view in just a few days. I'm enjoying myself. I like the people here. The nurses, half my age, are sweet and share with me their proposals with engagement rings sparkling. Others are tired mothers of toddlers who work night shifts with little sleep during the day. They all come with stories, and I try to memorize them. If I see them fully, they will see me as a patient worth taking care of with extra care. It works.

And then it happens. In the briefest of moments, I'm glad I have cancer. *What the actual fuck am I thinking?!* This is twisted, backward, maybe a result of the concoction of drugs that I'm on. Then it happens again. *This is nice: breakfast in bed, rest, no noise, no carpooling, long hours working, and running a household for six other humans.* Seriously, what is wrong with me?! Where is this coming from? No one in their right mind would be thankful for Leukemia. My heart beats faster; I'm so upset with my brain. I'm so upset with how I feel. I don't want to feel rested or enjoy my synthetic breakfast as much as I am.

But the truth is...my body loves this. My body, on a cellular level, is starting to fight cancer and heal before any chemotherapy treatments are even discussed. The air feels heavy. I pause, put my fork down, and sit silently, with a slight hum of hospital machines at my side. *Did I do this to myself? Did I live in a state of fight or flight longer than I can piece together? Did I say yes to everyone and everything else except for myself?* I did. I took advantage of the most authentic and most beautiful human being on the planet. I dragged it through mud, windstorms, and mountains made of jagged rocks. I kept pushing, kept driving, and never stopped to rest. My body was done with my disrespect, negligence, and dishonor toward the symphony of greatness and potential that I was blinded to.

I am convinced that my battle with Leukemia and my road to bone marrow transplant was not something that happened "to me." Leukemia is not a gene-embedded strand of DNA inherited from my great-aunt Rose, who died from a relentless fever and terrible body aches in 1812, with the cause of death unknown. It's not because I grew up near power lines. It's not because of what I choose to eat or

5

not eat. It's not because of weekend drinking or a short and stupid experiment with smoking. It's not because of a lack of sleep or exercise.

Leukemia didn't happen to me; I happened "to it." I chose my entire life to look past my simplest needs and meet the bigger needs of others. I decided never to see good as "good enough."

I chose to rely on the religious script and black-and-white rules to guide me through every decision in my life. I chose to stay in a loveless marriage where loneliness is at its peak when you're around each other rather than not. I chose to sacrifice everything I wanted to do and be for the sake of my five children.

Yes, that is what mothers do, but I did all these things to the extreme. Until one day, my body and immune system said, "You're done, and it's time to be reborn."

The following are 49 truths that I've learned through my continued rebirth. Life is too short to hold back raw emotions and words that make others uncomfortable, as they can bring healing and positive change.

I have nothing to lose here. I have been in the muddy trenches of battling through my mortality. I'm laying it all out on a table where Leukemia will never be welcome to sit again.

Acknowledgements

To Kyle, thank you for being my best friend through every step of this journey.

To my parents and in-laws, your devotion was endless. Thank you for driving hours at a moment's notice to manage all household duties, and for your fervent prayers and unwavering support.

To my sister, thank you for simply being by my side during my first chemotherapy treatment and for providing the most thoughtful care packages that brought comfort when I needed it most.

My brother, for your consistent prayers and encouraging texts that brightened my darkest days.

To the town of Point Pleasant, NJ—extended family, neighbors, cherished friends, and the dedicated community of Ocean Road School—your generosity in providing nightly meals for months was a consistent beacon of hope and practical support.

Dr. Tracey L. Ulshafer, my Guru and dear friend, thank you for expertly guiding me through the publication process. Beyond that, thank you for teaching me that 'everything is energy,' that I have the right to be here, and that I truly belong.

And to my precious children, Samuel Mark, Mollygrace Rose, Stella Noel, Charles Max, and Violet Kate, thank you for your trust and belief when I promised you I would be okay. It was your faith, combined with my knowing Christ had me firmly in His hands, that sustained me.

Dedication

Dedicated to my Mollygrace Rose –
The me I never allowed myself to be

" Our deepest fear is not that we are inadequate. Our deepest fear is that we are powerful beyond measure. It is our light, not our darkness, that most frightens us. We ask ourselves. Who am I to be brilliant, gorgeous, talented, fabulous? Actually, who are you not to be? You are a child of God. Your playing small does not serve the world. There is nothing enlightened about shrinking so that other people won't feel insecure around you. We are all meant to shine as children do. We were born to make manifest the glory of God that is within us. It's not just some of us; it's in everyone. And as we let our own light shine, we unconsciously give other people permission to do the same. As we are liberated from our own fear, our presence automatically liberates others."

- Marianne Williamson

I Choose…

I refuse to live in the caverns of pain and darkness.
I choose to see the light through the cracks.

I refuse to live in shame and regret.
I choose to see my ugly as a piece of art.

I refuse to hold back my fire to hide the glow.
I choose bravery.

I refuse to walk blindly through battles.
I choose tears and bloody wounds.

I refuse to acknowledge my inner critic.
I choose to stomp on the demon.

I refuse to keep quiet.
I choose to scream.

I refuse to hide lies and ugly truths.
I choose full exposure and judgment.

I refuse to make weakness my master.
I choose strength through tenacity.

I refuse to live life with anything but love.
I choose to make myself the most important person in the world.

I refuse to squash dreams to appease.
I choose adversity.

I refuse to stay in one place.
I choose to be uncomfortable.

I refuse to dishonor my body through unhealthy choices.
I choose conscious health.

I refuse to shame others to lift myself up.
I choose to embrace and forgive.

I refuse to numb the pain.
I choose to look in the mirror.

I refuse to stand on the edge.
I would rather fall and share the stories of my scars.

July 2022: Well This Sucks

It's 12:30 am on July 12th, 2022, and I am in the Emergency Room at Ocean Medical Center in Brick, NJ. My husband and oldest son arrived a few hours after me. Aside from an annoying pain I had been dealing with for a few weeks, there was a powerful whisper that seemed to suggest I should make the late-night drive.

A young doctor informs me that my pain is of no concern. Instead, the problem is that my blood counts are significantly "off." Whatever that means. I've been down similar roads like this before. Hard roads, long roads, and roads I wish no one ever had to travel. "No problem!" I consider myself one of those people who, when presented with "the hard things," understand I can handle it, and eventually, I do. Whatever it is, the doctors will figure it out, and I will get out of here.

I am moved from my makeshift room in the Emergency Room and am glad for that, as the gentleman next to me has been coughing for the past six hours and shared with his son on the phone that he was exposed to COVID last week. I'm transferred to a blue, synthetic leather, and well-worn wheelchair. It will serve as my transport to the hospital room where I have been admitted.

As I take a seat, I wonder how many people have sat in the same spot as I am now. What thoughts were running through their head? Did they have unanswered questions like I did? Did they think they were coming in for a peace-of-mind visit to learn that they would then be admitted? That's how my mind works; I've been accustomed to it for as long as I can remember. It goes like this. I have an idea, I learn something new, or I see something as mundane and as simple as an old wheelchair, and find that I'm not comfortable with the surface-based representation. There is always more to learn and even more to be curious about. There is a story behind something and someone always.

The nurse wheels me through the halls of the bustling ER. It's a busy night. Things seem to be running smoothly among the nurses and patients, and I find myself having pangs of jealousy when I see a man my age getting stitches on his knee. I want stitches on my knee. I don't want this. My husband and son walk with quiet yet confident footsteps behind me. My son seems to be more of a man to me than he ever was before. I feel safe with both of them. Two men, my strong support.

We take the elevator and ride it up one floor in silence. The doors open, and we turn right. Ahead of me is a long, white, pristine hospital corridor that lasts forever. I feel like I'm in a movie and transitioning to a scene that presents the plot twist. It is there that I feel it. It is there that I embody the inner knowing.

My entire being feels the certainty of knowing that my life will be abruptly stopping and restarting over the next few days. My brain takes a hundred snapshots of this smooth, white hallway before me. I don't see the end; I feel the beginning, and it's exactly here where I need to stay. I envision writing about this moment and wondering what words will follow. *"Stay present,"* I say to myself, *"Breathe,"* I say to myself, *"Trust the process." Stay present, breathe, and trust the process. Stay present, breathe, and trust the process.* I am a firm believer in affirmations. The power of our internal language can either bring forth health or illness.

17

I crawl into the uncomfortable hospital bed. I think about my five children and begin to plan the summer day to come. The day I naively believe I will be a part of. Earlier that day, I sat on the beach with them and took part in my favorite summer activity. Watching them. Watching my 7-year-old twins race one another on the beach, digging for sand crabs, and possibly discovering a sandbar in the distance if they were lucky enough.

I envy my older girls as they walk with ease to the shore, clothed in confidence and a surfboard in tow. I see their silhouettes as they sit on their boards in the distance, waiting for the next good wave. They catch them, some better than others, and return for more. It's in those moments that I know my children are content. They are present with the sand and the crabs, the ankle-deep sand bar water, and the next best wave to come. I don't take these moments for granted. I never have. I've relished from the very beginning when each 5-7lb. miracle was handed to me, and how quickly these years would go.

The next few days involve drawing blood samples. Hourly vitals are taken, and there is little time to sleep, as it seems there is a rush to find the answers. I keep a notepad at my bedside to record the names of each doctor I meet and the information they share. I carefully tape their business cards to the inside of a notebook, making me feel as though I'm in control of whatever chaos is taking place in my body.

I ask questions, and I study their body language carefully. When eye contact is not direct, I know information is being withheld for an uncertain diagnosis. When arms are folded, it's a sign of guarding their emotional state. When doctors choose to stand versus sit, it seems to be a way to detach themselves from an emotional

18

connection with their patients. My brain is flooded with blood count numbers and phrases like blood disorder, autoimmune disease, Lyme disease, and bone marrow abnormalities.

They share these terms to hide the diagnosis everyone fears the most, yet the one I've known has been there all along. I want to hear the word and face it with angst, anger, and motivation, just like I did at the start of every race I ran through middle school, high school, and college. I wanted to start what I feared the most.

On day three, a bone marrow biopsy was ordered. I don't know much about this procedure or what it tests for, but I know it is used to rule out serious blood deficiencies. I am tempted to Google the procedure and maybe even watch a YouTube video just because I can. In the end, I don't, and I'm glad.

The doctor is kind and gentle, and I envision him as a medical student years ago who silently observed the details of what he was being taught, worked hard, yet stayed out of the limelight. He assures me that the procedure is not as bad as most think. Just him sharing this tells me that many have had a bad experience, or it tells me that many aren't tough enough to handle it. I choose to believe the latter, and I believe that this is another challenge that I can overcome.

Difficult things or situations are only hard when you decide for them to be. We give more power than we deserve to the things that deplete us. I wonder why we don't do the same for things that motivate us. Why don't we feed the passions of what we excel at to the same level we give emotionally to the dentist appointment we dread? Emotion is energy, and energy is either uplifting or defeating. I find myself teetering on the balance beam of indecision regarding the impending bone marrow procedure. Should I fear it, or should I fight through it?

I lay on my side in my hospital bed and grip the bed rail with gentle ease. I know that if I grip too hard too soon, there will be nothing left to squeeze if I find myself in an unbearable place. A handsome young intern offers his hand for me to squeeze throughout the procedure as the doctor prepares the tools. His offering is another clue that this might not be the most pleasant experience. I'm annoyed with the intern because I can't tell if he's doing this to support me or impress his teacher with his bedside manner, my Doctor. I tell my brain to stop being so "judgy" and instead be grateful for human contact. I feel alone. I am alone. Like so many other times in my life, I find myself in this place of loneliness.

The procedure is taking a while. The doctor is trying a second time to retrieve my bone marrow as the first time; he makes cautious light of the fact that my bones are "too strong from all that yoga." I grip the bed rail as tightly as I can and watch the coloring of my fingertips change. I read the bracelet I bought at a local boutique five days earlier. "Keep Going." My other hand squeezes the intern's hand, and I'm thankful for him, even if he's trying to impress his teacher. After all, I would have done it as a student. I don't blame him. He's invested in his studies and wants nothing more than to someday administer this procedure confidently on his own.

A warm tear rolls so slowly down my cheek, and it tickles. I'm afraid to move my head to wipe it on the pillow. I'm trying to be as still as possible to get this moment over with. Somehow, the end arrives. I breathe air like I haven't breathed in the past 20 minutes. Once again, I hear the murmurings from others in the room. "Good job, you're brave; that wasn't easy." But to me, that's always been my walk. That's always been the sideline chatter to any difficult race I've run. I've found that so many things are not easy because easy things happen without you even realizing it.

Easy is choosing an area of study in college that bores you, but you know it will get you a job upon graduating. Easy is to stay in a relationship that feels more lonely when you are with the person than when you are without them. Easy is saying that someone else can do it better than you and, unfortunately, believing in that untruth. I don't choose easy often because easy doesn't change you. Easy numbs you and sedates the plethora and depth of every morsel of energy, talent, and idea hidden in the caverns of what makes you who you are. These things crave to be awakened not only for your growth but for the growth of others.

Hard is dealing with unfortunate situations you didn't see coming, and figuring out how to make the play that might ultimately save the game. Life-changing moments where your emotional response is either a tornado of restructuring your inner being or an earthquake that you somehow outrun, not to feel its true impact. But you feel it, beneath you, every day, the instability of something that used to feel steady yet too easy at the same time.

On July 15th, 2022, at 10:02 in the morning, a very kind Dr. sits at the end of my bed. Her medical students walk in close behind and stand along the wall as she prepares to share the final results of the frantic testing with me. I don't look at my doctor right away; instead, I look at the ones who I know are more vulnerable behind her. She has had a lot of practice disconnecting emotionally from her patients. She has to protect herself so that she can go home and laugh with her two-year-old and hug her husband.

The students are young, in their twenties. I like them and I don't even know them. All the signs are there. Gazes not meeting mine, slight fidgeting, pretending to be taking notes on iPads, and arms crossed, except for one. She wears glasses slightly too big for her face, but somehow they work. I'm jealous of her ginger hair in two braids and fly-away angel hairs around her forehead. Her white coat was buttoned, and her hands were folded neatly before her body. She takes her role as a medical student seriously. Her eyes meet mine, her face is stoic, and she stands in respect of the moment because she's not afraid to share the "hard" of this moment with me. I conclude, because of this, that she will be the best doctor of all of them.

My doctor wears a pristinely clear face guard and a K99 mask. Her eyes are bright, her skin is clear, and her figure is stunning. She exhibits grace, beauty, and intelligence, making her words float out gently. As she delivers the message, her tone is even, combining empathy and non-attachment.

"Sarah, I want you to look in my eyes and nowhere else. I want you to understand that the information I share with you in the next few moments will only be expanded upon by my fellow research team and the people standing behind me. You are not to Google, read articles, or seek to accept information from others who have walked the journey I am about to share with you. Sarah, our team of doctors has concluded through our various methods of testing that your bone marrow is producing blast cells that are consistent with a diagnosis of Acute Myeloid Leukemia with mutation."

My head immediately begins to feel a slight buzzing sound. I look to my left and see Kyle drop his head as if nothing could hold it up. I am glad that the serendipity of his being there for a short visit allowed him to hear this news as well. I was in my body for a brief moment.

In the moments following, I found myself floating just outside of the 44-year-old woman sitting cross-legged on the end of her hospital bed with her blue gown unbuttoned in the back because she refused to believe she was staying in the hospital much longer. I look at how her back is arched forward and how her shoulders shake as she begins to cry. She doesn't know why she's crying because she knows she's not going to die. She knows she won't fail, and it's not a defeat. She cries because she hopes she has enough fight for the toughest battle yet.

She pretends to take in the words of her doctor, but instead envisions what Leukemia would look like if it were a monster. She cries because she is angry at this monster who has no right to be messing with her. She cries because she is required once again to push through, fall, bleed, and scream through a storm that will likely be the most unpredictable and, at times, unbearable hours of her life. She cries because she knows it's the closest thing to feeling anything she can at the moment, even if that *anything* is nothing she can yet define.

Truth 1: You are the Most Important Person

It's not a selfish way of thinking; it's a survival way of thinking.

One of the things that has always impressed me about kids is their unwavering devotion to who they are. No one else in the world matters except for themselves. They are terrible listeners who only think about what they want to say. They want to be first in line or the fastest runner in their grade. They are boosted with confidence by any compliment, though they don't naturally think of giving a compliment. They make choices based on how the outcome might positively affect them. They think of themselves and only themselves, believing they are the most important person. As adults, we sometimes cater to this, but at the same time, we understand that they are growing and learning, and will eventually develop a more balanced perspective on the world and their place in it.

It's been my experience that the older we get, the less important we feel. We look outside ourselves for validation, compliments, a boss affirming us, or a teenager just wanting to spend time with us. We are conditioned to think we are unimportant because something else or someone else is more important. We ignore that tiny voice that says, "You matter, and you are worth it."

The truth is simple. You ARE the most important person in this world. It's not a selfish way of thinking; it's a survival way of thinking. We survive with food, water, clothing, shelter, sex, and relationships. However, if we only seek these things for survival and do not validate who we are and our needs on a daily basis, we are slowly disintegrating from the inside out. What gets you excited? What is something you want to learn? Where is a place you want to travel to? What is it that feeds your unique soul? When we pause and ask ourselves these questions, many of us struggle to find immediate answers.

I've led hundreds of workshops regarding self-care, self-worth, and self-identity. I encouraged my listeners to remember who they were before they were teachers, wives, husbands, or parents. Most of them look at me blankly, which I chalk up to them thinking they didn't have time for my bull-shit pep talk. That was okay with me as I knew I was planting a seed. But others cocked their heads a bit, uncrossed their arms, and began scratching down notes. My message was simple: "Find the things that excite you, make you happy, and make you feel that you are important without external validation!"

After presenting to a group of exhausted-looking high school teachers at a Tuesday faculty meeting they didn't want to attend, a teacher approached me. She approached me, and I liked her because she was one of the few who didn't have the laptop open, pretending to pay attention to my message. I get it. I'm a teacher. Time is limited, and content at faculty meetings is always back-burner information. Her eyes were teary, and I could tell she wanted to choose just the right words to share with me. She was looking at me as if I were a superior. I hate that. Just because I'm a presenter doesn't mean I'm wiser or more intelligent than anyone attending my workshops. Her body language softened when I smiled. She paused, searching for words. She looked at me and said, " I have a story to tell, but I've never felt important enough for others to want to hear it."

25

We talked for a while, and naturally, I encouraged her to start writing. To write anything and everything she feels. I shared with her that the opinions and reactions of others do not matter. What matters is that she honors the voice inside her that encourages her to begin fulfilling this calling. What I expect to happen is that she discovers how important she is and how important her story is while she is writing. I hope she sees herself beyond the societal labels that have defined her.

The magic that takes place when we begin to see ourselves as important starts to shift the energy around us and within us. Naturally, we are drawn to others who share our values, confidence, and self-worth. This newly discovered energy propels us to pull back from those who drain the truth of our importance. It's liberating to detach from relationships we've held onto for far too long, keeping the peace within the other person, rather than honoring the peace our bodies desperately desire.

I have worked through this process of relationship pruning and continue to do so. It's not easy, but it's also not my responsibility to be concerned about the other person's well-being if they negatively affect mine. The result is liberating, and the shift you feel internally is powerful. When you honor who you are and honor your specific needs, opportunities begin to flood as you create space for who you are meant to be. You no longer need to be defined by someone else's view of you. And that truth brings us back to the mindset of a child. Be selfish and believe that, above all others in this entire world, you are the one who matters the most. Does this mean you try to get as much as you can at the expense of others, or tune out the opinions of others? Not at all. Instead, this is an internal recognition that, when discovered, can allow you to blossom and grow with every pruned realization you consciously make.

I recently took a new job as a Kindergarten teacher in my local school district. As I type these words, I see colorful art projects on the wall, tiny chairs, and an array of homemade pictures my littles have gifted me. I haven't taught in 20 years, so I felt somewhat unprepared for this new position. The day before I started the job, a friend texted me a phrase we had all heard over a hundred times, but it made more sense this time than ever. "Don't try to reinvent the wheel." I applied this immediately to my fears and have this phrase taped to my desk as a daily reminder to do only what I need to do now. Good is good enough.

I've lived my whole life overthinking. I looped through thought after thought. Analyzing and creating Venn Diagrams in my head and pro/con lists on notepads. The mental energy required was exhausting, and my body became accustomed to living in a state of unrest and confusion. In some ways, I felt more comfortable with indecision than with a decision. Now, post-cancer, I don't overthink. I live consciously and make choices based on what my body tells me is true and right. It takes a second to react, yet it takes a moment to respond.

I live in the moment now. My body has spent years reacting and living in a state of unconscious mayhem where all kinds of wheels are trying to be reinvented simultaneously. To the point that halfway through the process, I would forget what I was trying to invent. Our heads get in the way. We think they help, but they don't. Ask yourself, "Does this decision, relationship, or situation serve my overall well-being?" If the answer is "no," then you have your answer.

Don't go back and forth; don't be tempted to go down the rabbit trail of "what-ifs and buts." You ARE the most important person, and your body knows that. Your mind is always the one trailing behind, needing to be constantly and consciously reminded.

I've learned over and over again through these past 16 months post my diagnosis that my health is entirely dependent upon the choices I make in favor of furthering my development into the best human I can be, not for anyone else but for me. When you embrace the not selfish mentality of mattering and owning all of who you are (even the ugly parts), you make space to grow into the parts waiting for you. And that's the exciting part of all of this self-work! There are gifts, relationships, and opportunities waiting just around the corner for you. However, this depends on how much energy you invest in yourself and how much you prioritize your own needs.

My body had had enough, and it caved from the inside out. I was trying so hard for so many years to reach my full potential, but I snuffed it out to serve the needs of others, and I chose to hang out with my brain on the back burner instead.

Without going into too much scientific or medical detail, Leukemia is simply the breakdown of one's immune system. My core defenses, down to a cellular level, began to fail me. These cells were shut down, muted, and unrecognized for their entire life. I am entirely okay confessing that I chose this disease; it didn't choose me. Medical experts will disagree with me, and you might think this is an overly simplistic view regarding one of the deadliest cancers out there. But that doesn't matter. What matters is that I know this truth and believe it. I am well aware that it will enable me to make decisions based on whether my sensory and cellular systems are adequately nourished.

The bottom line is that you already know all the answers. There's no need to allow your head to get too involved. Get silent. Pause. Your sensory system has the answer. It's just up to you whether or not you want to trust the part of you that knows you are the most important person in the room.

Truth 2: Don't Hide Your Pain

However, I eventually understood that the energy it took to hide the pain became more exhausting than the energy to start feeling it.

Mrs. Brown's Kindergarten class was the quintessential storybook classroom you would expect to see in 1984. Desks lined neatly in rows, big and simple Alphabet letters taped along the top of the chalkboard, and blow-up letter people scattered around the room. The week's highlight was finding the week's letter person on Monday. And since the classroom was minimal with "stuff," it was easy to spot the creepy-looking creatures hiding behind the play kitchen that served as the golden gate of playtime.

I kept to myself amidst the bustle of five-year-old fun and noise. I colored within the lines and was careful not to press too hard on my paper so that I wouldn't make a hole. I knew Mrs. Brown liked me because I felt it from her. She didn't have to tell me I was important. I just knew. And that's what makes a good teacher—holding space for your students in an environment where, if they don't trust you, there is no reason for them to learn or produce a positive outcome for you.

I trusted and wanted to please her, but I also wanted to do everything well. I was not a hand-raiser and continued not to be a hand-raiser through high school. Mrs. Brown knew this and didn't call on me out of surprise because she realized it would do more emotional harm to a student like me than it was worth. My face would flush, I would freeze, and any academic answer at that point wasn't worth the increase in my heart rate. She knew I was understanding the content, as my work reflected that. She knew I was socially adapted to her classroom because I had no problem playing the big sister role in the kitchen or running around playing "Cooties" on the playground. However, all the structure and quiet I had set up for myself sometimes worked against me. I became used to hiding behind my ideas, two neat braids, and cotton dresses with white collars, so much so that I thought I should hide the pain.

It must have been early September or sometime in June. The classroom was hot. The lights were low, and the ceiling fans were on full blast. I was working quietly, as was the entire class. Mrs. Brown was in front of the classroom, making me feel safe. Suddenly, I feel a pinch in the upper part of my dress. It alarms me, and it hurts. I wince, and I freeze. It happens again. This time, the pain is sharp, shooting, and familiar. It happens two more times in quick succession. I peek through the lace collar of the dress and see a wasp. It's black and awful-looking. I don't know what to do. Maybe it will fly away on its own, and then I can get through the misery without a scene or attention. The last thing I want to have happen is for my classmates to see me cry. I feel my body get tense, my face hot, and I'm stuck there in a mental battle of needing help or absorbing the pain and hoping it will dissolve or fly away on its own.

I can't focus on my work, and I can't find the strength to hold back my tears. Once the first tear fell, the others followed quickly, as if in anger. I didn't let them out with the first sting. Mrs. Brown sees me, but she doesn't say anything. Instead, she puts her hand on my shoulder and leads me outside the classroom with the door slightly cracked behind her. I breathe; I'm safe now. She's on the larger side but finds me important enough to squat down next to me. We solve the problem together by taking care of the wasp. I melt into her chest, and she hugs me while I cry. I'm physically sore, emotionally exhausted, and relieved at the same time. I don't remember what she said to me. But I remember how she made me feel. I felt protected and safe. I felt I was the only person who mattered to her at that moment. She took on the emotional pain I could not carry on my own. And more importantly, created space for me to practice my first big lesson of vulnerability.

Thirty-two years later, I'm driving myself to the Emergency room on a rainy Sunday morning in January. I'm 20 weeks pregnant, and something is not right. I show no signs of bleeding, backaches, or preterm labor. Instead, a "knowing" and for the sake of assurance, I need to confirm that all is okay. Just last week, I felt the flutterings of my baby kicking, but not this week.

I'm in a tiny room waiting for a nurse to get a doppler to appease me. She seems annoyed that I'm here with no apparent signs of alarm. She assumes I'm some anxious, type-A mom who will probably be back in two weeks, asking to hear the heartbeat again. I don't care what she thinks. I am wise and old enough to know that trusting that still-small voice rules out any judgment from those outside my "knowing."

She sits on the side of my bed after hurriedly smearing cold jelly on the wand. I wince when she begins to glide it across my belly. A part of her likes knowing I'm a bit uncomfortable, as her body language exudes annoyance that she's having to do this. Seconds later, we hear a heartbeat.

I sigh with relief. She doesn't. She cocks her head and moves the wand to different positions on my belly. The heartbeat continues to march forward in the same rhythm, but now a bit faster. I keep expecting her to wrap things up, but she doesn't. I tell her how relieved I am that all is okay. She looked at me and said, "Honey, that's your heartbeat." She wheels me to an ultrasound room to get a better look at things. I already know. I don't need an ultrasound. The air is heavy, it's still raining outside, and everything in my body feels like death. The radiologist thinks she's sly when she slightly turns the screen away from me. She's quiet, and the room feels extra small and dark. The click-click sound of pictures taken from every angle possible finally ends.

I wait, Kyle arrives, and I cry. The Doctor comes in. Anything he plans to say, I can already feel in his energy. But I will never forget the exact words. When trauma is created in the body, the subconscious clings to the emotion, and we hold tighter to these memories than the ones filled with joy. He takes a breath, places his hands behind his back, and lowers his chin. "Mrs. Stevenson, there is no movement consistent with a 20-week-old fetus." It took him all of 12 seconds to deliver this news. He stood stoically and poised, offering minimal condolences. I knew that as soon as he stepped out of the room, he would be on to his following scan to get home to his family sooner. I was left with a heaviness I had never felt before. This heaviness was death. My body was embodying death.

Since I was too far along in the pregnancy, the only way for the baby to be taken care of was through birth. I shuddered at the thought and, worse, at the picture I was creating in my mind. The doctor offered to admit me right then. I immediately said, "No, I need one more night with my baby." I don't know where the words came from; they

33

just came. Maybe it was morbid of me to keep a dead baby within me one more day, but to me, that was my baby who, at one time, had a heart that beat below my own. I went to bed before Kyle so I could cry myself to sleep. I held my belly and anxiously poked around to feel my baby's small structures.

The birth was not unto life but unto death. Guttural screams came from a place deep and dark through every labor pain released as my little boy slid limply into the world. He is swept away and returns wrapped in a tiny, tan blanket that volunteers knit for babies like mine. The blanket smells like a mixture of sterile hospital chemicals and baby powder. A quick ceremony is conducted. My nurse reads the 23rd Psalm from her bible, and I recite the words with her. Her voice quivers a bit as she reads. This comforts me because it means she is feeling his loss, and that honors that he was a human to her, too. I watch my baby leave the room in the arms of that same nurse. I sink into a darkness I didn't know existed.

The following weeks involved enrolling my three-year-old in preschool in mid-January, as I couldn't imagine jumping back into being a "fun" stay-at-home mom. I want no one around. I closed the blinds and turned off the lights when the kids went to school. I don't answer the door when people drop off meals or flowers, and I ignore all phone calls. I sat under blankets on the couch, used frozen packs of vegetables on my aching, milk-filled breasts, and watched sad movies like "Steel Magnolias" so that I could keep crying. Crying felt good when no one was around. I could marinate in my pain without anyone interrupting the process. People try to offer comforting words, but I don't accept them. I'm too raw, I ache too deeply, and I'm annoyed that they have no idea how badly this hurts. And how awful it was to feel a life release like jello from your womb. That feeling is deeply embedded within me. Like a fossil never to be unetched, it gives me chills whenever I allow myself to revisit it. I'm offered bible verses that might help me get through the heartache. I smile and nod while burning inside with disgust at the ignorance of those offering "help." In retrospect, I see the intent, and I recognize how deeply I was hurt. I wasn't in a place to receive it. I was basking in self-preservation. Staying away from everyone made me feel in control, less vulnerable, and safe.

I worked hard to hide the pain of losing my baby boy. However, I eventually understood that the energy it took to hide the pain became more exhausting than the energy to start feeling it. I Google search a therapist in my area and start opening up to trusted friends. I enrolled in a 200-hour Yoga Teacher Training program to create a safe space for myself to work through the ache of loss. What follows is the discovery of a word that has now become and will always be my favorite word in the human language. Vulnerability. According to Brené Brown, Vulnerability is *"uncertainty, risk, and emotional exposure."* I wasn't sure how others would respond if I shared my ache. It was risky to wait for their response. And most importantly, I felt emotionally stripped down.

I delivered a dead baby. His name was Magnus William after his maternal grandfathers. He was 20 weeks old. I donated his body to research, and I have a custom-made Christmas stocking with the name Max on it from Pottery Barn.

I say it; I wait, breathe, and practice handling the responses that float my way.

I accept some and reject others. And what I discovered through this process is something I never saw coming. People I'm hardly close with start sharing about their depression, their broken marriages, their loneliness, and their teenagers who have been struggling with addiction. The list is endless. But their list is only being shared with me because I chose to share a piece of my list first. Sharing my ache creates a beautiful emotional transference with the other person. It creates space for that person to practice vulnerability. And it's not to one-up each other's pain. Their pain is no greater or smaller than my pain. It's all pain, and pain is never to be measured.

When we knowingly or unknowingly hide emotional pain, we will have no choice but to sit in the stings over and over again. The wasp won't leave; it taunts, bruises, and teases you. You will create a hard shell and disguise yourself behind flashy Facebook posts, expensive boats, and an "I'm fine" response to anyone who asks how you're doing. I've lived that way for far too long and suffered the consequences of breaking down my immune system to a point where it gave up on me.

The beauty in exposing the pain and the parts of you that you hide becomes the stepping stone to who you were meant to be. Not only do you give others a safe space to share their ache, but you begin to honor your body and your entire being. You start to heal and eventually understand that the more shit you expose, the lighter you feel. (No pun intended!) With every ugly truth released, you start peeling back tiny layers of your true version. We are comfortable living in the lie versions of ourselves. Because that's self-protection, we think it's easier, but it's not. We are held by invisible chains made of the strongest steel.

Share your mistakes and own them: I lied to my children, and I deeply regret it.

Share your pain and feel the release: I gave birth to a dead baby. His name was Magnus William Stevenson.
Share your trauma and heal: At age 19, I was raped and lived in the lie that it was my fault.

Share the parts of yourself that disgust you and shame you: I was bulimic for ten years. I stole money from people to support my habit and stole hundreds of dollars worth of food from grocery stores and mini-marts.

Share your deepest fear: I will always be alone.

All of these things feel big because you allow them to be. They are wasps that are either released or trapped, capable of causing increasingly more damage. I give myself no excuses for the above confessions. That's who I am. And as I've said before, I have no reason to hide my truths anymore. When you dabble with death like I have, you realize that living in truth gives you life. The lies are what began the process of killing me.

Truth 3: Good is Good Enough

Striving and surpassing is a clever way to stuff down the shame we unknowingly embed in our DNA.

If you are an avid or competitive runner, you are well aware of what the two letters "PR" stand for. Personal Record. These two letters are a blessing and a curse when it comes to the sport. They represent a goal to strive for to produce a faster mile time, 5K time, or marathon time. They bring momentary feelings of elation when the former PR has been beaten, even if just by half a second. It doesn't sound like much, but to a 200-meter sprinter, that half a second is a well-deserved reward for dedicated training. And then there's the disappointment, self-loathing, and internal criticism of shame that confidently takes over when the PR is not achieved. And again, if that PR is half a second less, you enjoy it for a fleeting moment until you set your sights on the next race ahead.

Depending on the athlete, a list of "shoulds" rears its ugly head. I should have gone to bed earlier the night before the race, tapered more efficiently, trained harder, eaten better, weighed less, and so on. Not all athletes get in their heads with this kind of language, but I was adept at making the "should list" part of my daily script.

I was a three-season runner through high school and continued my love-hate relationship with running via a partial college scholarship. I wouldn't say I liked the sport because of the physical demands and the pressure to weigh less, train harder, and run faster. I loved the sport because of my teammates. But ultimately, when it came to the sport itself, I despised it. It had so much control over me; good was never good enough. I learned early that someone would always be faster than me, which I was okay with. I also learned that someone will always be thinner and stronger than me, which I was not OK with. That was an element of the sport that I could control. The numbers on the scale were easier to manipulate than the PR time for my next 5k.

I launched myself into the throes of a serious eating disorder throughout my entire college career. I believed the lie that I would be better than "good enough" if I lost weight and trained harder. Some races proved my reasoning, but some races confirmed I was a pathetic and secret bulimic who considered myself an athlete. I felt like a fraud. I felt like someone else should have been gifted the scholarship. I felt like I would never be better than good. I wanted to be the best version of myself, but I had no fucking clue where to begin. Pounding tubs of ice cream and packages of Oreos stuffed down the emotional pain to numb the lie that I was worth nothing and would never even be good enough.

I carried this lie through most of my marriage and parenting. I had to be better than good at these roles, or else I might fail. Secret PRs I set for myself included being physically available for my husband, even when I didn't want to be—scheduling date nights and ski trips in hopes it would save an already hopeless marriage. I hosted as many parties, picnics, and church gatherings as possible to prove to myself (not others) that I was better than good. I actively participated in Mom's groups, class mom, and a short and tiring few years of homeschooling. I was so busy striving for life PRs that I didn't realize I was sacrificing my physical life with every date on the calendar and commitment I didn't want to take. I was not honoring who I was. I was too afraid to stare into my partner's face and tell him I was not in love with him and hadn't been for a long time. I faked it. Stuffing down emotional pain, not through food, but instead through tasks and to-do lists. I believed that the failing marriage was all my fault.

Bottom line. Good is good enough. Life's PRs aren't for anyone but yourself. Your body and mind constantly remind you that you are a success. It's whether or not you choose to believe this or choose to feed the voice that whispers you can be half a second faster.

Why do we need perfection, PRs, and recognition so badly? It's because of the deep and dark valleys within us that we dare to look at due to the fear of what might come up. Striving and surpassing is a clever way to stuff down the shame we unknowingly embed in our DNA daily. Striving to be good at whatever you do, think, or say is always where you need to be. And even more importantly, accepting that you will fail, disappoint, and be so far off from your PR that you will forget the original PR you were trying to beat. But in time, you will find that PRs are nothing more than life's lie and that you must do everything according to the script you write for yourself.

People don't care or observe your actions or inactions as much as you think they do. The only people anyone cares about are themselves. Don't waste emotional or physical energy to prove who you are. You already know who you are. It just takes some self-study to get there eventually.

Your physical body wants to know and be affirmed that it is doing a good job for you. Anything beyond doing a good job is ego. It's pushing the limits. It's asking your body to dip into the reserves it has gotten used to repeatedly emptying. A car will go without an updated oil change just to be faithful to the owner. But there will be a moment when that car can't go one more mile. It won't want to fail; it just won't have a choice. I sat in the reserve tank of my body for years until my body stopped running for me.

When I was in first grade, my teacher suggested to my parents that I start playing the board game "Perfection." This game challenged the player to place all the plastic puzzle pieces in the corresponding spots before the buzzer went off, causing the entire board to release all that I had worked to solve. As a seven-year-old, this was an agonizing and stressful game. At any moment, the board could pop. My time and effort would hold no value. I would only be successful if I were perfect.

I took my time as a student. I was an over-thinker, which got in the way of production. So, being handed the game of perfection meant that I was far from perfect and taught me that it was more important to produce than to feel. According to Mrs. G's first-grade expectations, being good at something was not good enough. Perfection was the goal, but for what reason?

As a teacher, I don't judge her for her choice of strategy. She was doing the best she knew how at the moment. She saw a little girl who was quiet, reserved, and reflective. All of which got in the way of keeping up with the rest of the class. In my six-year-old brain, I now falsely believed that things weren't good unless they were perfect. I responded to life's small and big challenges based solely on whether or not I would come out better than good. But the ironic part is that there is no measure for personal perfection, and outsiders watching your life don't care how good you are at something.

We are the only ones deciding how much energy we want to waste on something that might harm us more than help us. Do you need to volunteer for that school committee? Do you need to run for the school board office, or do you want to? Do you need to host Thanksgiving dinner, or would someone else be able to do it? Do you need to ensure all five food groups are on the table for dinner, or can you slide by with grilled cheese or cereal one night? Do you need to buy a house outside of your budget so that you can relish in the faces of friends who walk through your doors? The list goes on and on and on.

We unknowingly seek perfection, but it takes emotional courage to feel content knowing that good is good enough. Your body wants good. It doesn't like the pressure of the endless PRs we place on ourselves. After a while, your body won't trust you anymore. After a while, you will become tired and disillusioned with the expectations that will only lead to anger and exhaustion.

From now on, I live with the "good is good enough" mantra. I have nothing to prove to anyone and everything to gain by extending more extraordinary grace and emotional support to myself. My prior need for constant PRs dipped into the reserve of any immunity I had left to fight off infection. My body gave up. It could no longer trust its owner.

I am the most important person in the room, and you, my friend, are the most important person in *your* room. You are perfect because you are good enough.

Truth 4: Change It

The truth in our dreams rests in trusting ourselves and what the outcome could be instead of what we think the outcome will be.

A friend of mine got me into the stairmaster at the gym. We have a 10-minute love-hate relationship, where I give myself mini pep talks and try not to look at the minutes that have passed. I do this machine because it's a challenge, and I do it because anything that stares you in the face as a challenge also requires discipline. This particular morning, I looked out on the gym floor and scanned the people, the faces, the interactions, and the subtleties of human interaction. At 5:47 a.m., most people looked tired. They stay in their lane mostly. They are sticking to the machines and movements they've refined over the years. They always have the same routine, rarely deviating from what they feel is the best workout.

And then the questions struck me. Why are all these people doing the same thing every day? Why am I doing mostly the same thing? Why does everyone seem to be stuck in the "sameness " routine? The crazy part is that we don't know we are doing this. Myself included! I tend to stick to the same exercises, yoga routines, and 12 minutes of sauna time each day. I watch these strangers and conclude that at one point in their lives, they had a dream, a vision, something they looked toward and maybe even worked at until whispered lies of defeat set in. Maybe they even tasted some of their dreams before fear set in, insecurities, self-doubt, or even worse, "I'm not worthy."

The truth in our dreams rests in trusting ourselves and what the outcome *could be* instead of what we think the outcome will be. We put up stop signs, create traffic jams, and end up at too many police checkpoints along our individual roads. And when we feel like we are getting somewhere, we fall back on good old self-sabotage techniques. *Why?* Because we don't feel worthy. We look to the ones who have gone before us. They seem to have figured it out pretty quickly. *Good for them,* we say to ourselves. We admire them, want to be them, and get jealous of them. The bottom line is that it's easier to sit on the sidelines and judge the plays rather than be in the huddle and figure it out. And by the way, no one knows what they are doing.

I am convinced that much of my blood-borne illness resulted from one word. Refuse. I refused to leave a marriage that crushed my spirit instead of making it grow. I refused to return to work full-time because, as I believed, "good moms" stay home with their toddlers. I refused to challenge others' opinions because I didn't want them to feel bad. I refused to say no to making coffee cakes for church bake sales because I didn't want to put another tired mom out. I refused to take a day off from the gym because that meant I might be lazy. I refused to say no to everything that, over time, melted my fire-centered self.

The fire eventually burned down to cinders and then dissolved into ash. And you will only become ash when you live to appease others and refuse to see yourself as the most powerful being on the planet. And there is nothing to do with ash other than to throw it out and make way for someone else's fire to take over the pit.

How do we fix this fucked up, patterned behavior? The first step is to recognize when our body falls into appeasement mode. And you can start small. I have an exercise you can practice, which I would like to call the "drive-through challenge." The next time you find yourself in the Starbucks drive-through line, put aside what you "think" you should order or what you order regularly. Instead, order something that you "want" to order. Take a look at the glossy pictures of cake pops, frothy lattes, panini sandwiches, cookies, and brownies. Order what you want! Start by honoring the simplest of pleasures: food and drink. Then, pull into an empty parking space and sip that 600-calorie drink slowly. Eat the brownie with your eyes closed and chew slowly. Make love to the food, and you fall in love with a little piece of yourself. I am not suggesting you do this every time you find yourself in your favorite fast food line. Do this when the desire strikes you.

Listen to what your body needs on a cellular level. Listening with cellular ears versus cognitive ears are two entirely different means of awareness. When you make a mental choice, it is based on a series of information that most of us consider repeatedly. When you make an immediate choice on a cellular level, whether you like the answer or not, the answer is there. It is there that we can begin to practice the power of change. To practice it, we have to accept the answer for what it is.

Your body wants to change. It constantly tells you what it wants to change. But we stuff down the nagging voice and replace it with what we think is better. I never wanted to leave a marriage. I didn't. I didn't stand on an altar on July 21, 2001, to envision a divorce 22 years later. I didn't expect to break the hearts of my five children or navigate life alone. But as years passed and as my heart became

45

heavier, my days became longer, and I felt less and less loved, I thought I could be strong enough to push through the ache of what I thought I would have. I grieve the loss of a long life with a partner that I was once in love with, but I don't grieve the toll that the relationship took on my health. I should have left my marriage twelve years ago, but I didn't have the strength. I thought the cognitive part of my brain could heal the deepening wounds through more date nights, getaways, therapy appointments, and family day trips. Inside, my body was craving change. I knew I would better serve my overall well-being if I just listened. But I didn't want to disappoint and let down the five little hearts under my roof. Little did I know... they wanted the change too. My teens saw a woman they had once admired as strong, but who was now pretending to be strong, which is worse than being weak.

My oldest son and I would take the 40-minute drive north every Friday and Saturday to work together at a five-star restaurant for two years. I served fancy cocktails with dirty ice on the side and memorized specials that required me to practice pronunciation before presenting the costly dishes. He bussed, was a food runner, and ate as many free truffle fries as possible. We worked well together, and though we didn't always enjoy the dynamic, we knew we were building something that we could look back upon as "good" for years to come.

Our shifts usually ended around 12:30 am. I would drive home barefoot as my feet were so sore. He would melt into reflection mode in the passenger seat and recall the crazy scenarios. We would laugh about drunk patrons, messed up food orders, cooks clearly on drugs, and co-workers who were challenging to work with. He would talk my ear off the entire ride home, and I loved every minute.

One night, in particular, he was quiet. I knew he was thinking about something, but I didn't pry. When you question a teenager, you often get the opposite reaction you hoped for. You get shut-down mode. Handling teens is like carrying a martini glass on a small tray without spilling it. Eyes ahead, thumb on the glass, don't think, tread lightly. "Mom, why are you still in this?" At first, I had no idea what he was referring to. He continues to reflect and share how he can see and feel the disconnect between me and his father. He continues, "Are you and Dad okay?" I let my guard down. I told him I was unhappy and depressed, working as much as I could because his father wouldn't make up for what our family needed. He was quiet, and I was making the first steps toward my way out. I had unveiled to my oldest child that a divorce was on the horizon. Our ride home was quiet after that. The quietest it had ever been.

When you release what doesn't serve you, you will make a gateway to relationships and experiences that will. My marriage was a stopgap to my happiness. Fake it till ya make it. It rarely works when applied to a relationship, because it involves the heart. Don't mess with your heart. It will never forgive you. It only knows how to serve you, celebrate you, and promote you. Closing the door on your heart, refusing to change what doesn't align with what you envision as your best life, will lead to patterned behaviors, such as replicating the same 13 exercises every morning at 5:14 am for the avid Type-A gym-goer.

Truth 5: The Valleys of Vulnerability

When practiced, vulnerability negates fear and lies about self-worth, propelling connection and relational growth.

My love for words started in my 6th-grade Spanish class. Like any middle school language class, it's all about memorization and stringing together simple phrases. Of all the words I learned that year, the one that caught my tongue the most was "lechuga." It means lettuce. A dull, simple, no-substance word, but I loved to say it. It looked strong when I wrote it down, and I liked how it sounded when I said it. Nothing else stuck with me from my few years of language classes, but I was drawn to this word for whatever reason.

Not all words are this way. We avoid some because we know there is emotional accountability associated with them. Lechuga was not one of those words, unless I'm missing some weird psychological connection with lettuce from my childhood.

I didn't think much about the word vulnerability for most of my life. It wasn't until I started researching this topic for the hundreds of student assemblies and staff professional development workshops I led during my six-year stint as a Social and Emotional Learning Consultant. I didn't breach this topic until I had spent a few years earning the trust of the educators present. It's not an easy topic for people to relate to because we don't want to be vulnerable. We don't want to be vulnerable even to ourselves. Fortunately, I was given opportunities through a few districts that were willing to reinstate my services on a year-to-year basis. This worked beautifully because presenting on any topic of self-awareness, self-regulation, and self-study was certainly not a one-time deal. The schools I saw as most successful in their commitment to my agenda of building a stronger social environment among staff and students were those that recognized the value in consistency.

I grew up in a home founded in a faith that didn't encourage the ugly side of vulnerability, which I have since seen as beautiful. A less aggressive side of vulnerability was "allowed" or accepted. It was okay to share financial struggles and ask for prayer. It was OK to share marital problems and ask for prayer. It was OK to share a battle with addiction and ask for prayer. It was okay to share a struggle with depression and ask for prayer. Yes, these are significant areas of vulnerability for some people, but they aren't what I like to call the "deep valley vulnerability" topics. It also seemed that the fallback of "prayer" was the allowance people relied upon to share. I saw right through the clever cover-up and wondered why people can't just share the hard stuff. Why did it always have to be hidden behind the guise of prayer?

I learned quickly that I was allowed to share shades of vulnerability, but only if it didn't come out too ugly or, even worse, cause shame to my parents. I had to protect their image as church leaders, youth group facilitators, and active parents in the school district. So, I lived behind my curtain of self-protection and allowed the play of shame to follow the script. It was constantly running in the back of my brain. There was no intermission; the scene changed without a chance to breathe. I wanted to share with the audience the darker aspects of my life. But fear was unknowingly attached to every thought. The lie that followed was that I would not be accepted. My view of Christ was so conflicted. I couldn't equate his love for me, his love for sinners, and his infinite amount of grace. I didn't feel safe with the God I served.

During my early adult years, I was mostly caught up in the throes of the monster that held me down with chains and dictated every next step, word, action, or thought I had. Calorie counting, hours of daily workouts, purging up to twenty times a day, and loads and loads of self-loathing alone in my single college dorm room.

I remember once attending a short seminar in one of the girls' dormitories concerning eating disorders. The woman who presented was strong and independent, and she shared candidly about how difficult it was to shake the beast and conquer something that had stolen too many days of her life. I'm assuming this seminar was the college's way of supporting the silent suffering like myself. I sat there in awe of her, admired her, but mostly was jealous of her. I knew at the time that this was irrational. I hated that she was in a place of vulnerability.

I hated that she exuded such a feminine confidence about herself. I hated myself for the thoughts I was projecting. I imagined being self-aware and confident like her someday. However, being only 19, I did not have a very realistic mental picture of myself, either in the present or the future. I wanted to stay after the 30-minute presentation and sit next to her. I didn't know what I would ask her or what we would talk about. I just wanted to be in her presence. Someone who could feel the deep valley of vulnerability in my brain without me having to say any words.

I was on the precipice of walking up to her when the presentation was over. It was a three-minute mental battle that involved drawing pictures of Venn diagrams, making a pro and con list, and asking, "What if I do v. what if I don't talk to her?" I knew that on that entire college campus, there was one person that I might be able to trust with my "ugly," and that person was just ten feet away. But fear pulled down the curtain, and the scenes got worse in my brain. I couldn't find the courage to be vulnerable. I went back to my room, binged on vending machine candy bars, threw up, and went to bed with swollen glands and puffy eyes.

Vulnerability is not something any of us are comfortable with. Ask someone what it looks like to be vulnerable, and watch them squirm. Likely, they won't give you a definition sufficient to its meaning. This isn't because they are skirting around the topic. Instead, they are unaware of the role it plays in daily life choices and relationships.

When practiced, vulnerability negates fear and lies about self-worth, propelling connection and success. We are all afraid of exposing who we are. We mask our ugly through expensive clothes, over-the-top vacations, and mortgages we can't afford. We figure that if we create enough of a materialistic barrier, we won't be challenged to expose our true selves. However, the problem with these temporary barriers is that when life hits hard and takes an unexpected turn, these "things" we think can hide our pain only make it worse. We become so accustomed to not feeling and being fake that we don't know how to feel when we are challenged. And there, the addiction begins to get stronger. Buy more stuff, drink more alcohol, binge longer, work harder, make more money. Your body is screaming to be heard. It's tired of being suffocated through temporary addictions that falsely define us. Something amazing happens when you start practicing sharing who you are. People listen. They pause and may not respond much, but it's enough for them to be curious about the risk you took in trusting them with some heavy emotional energy.

Not everyone wants to hear it; you can figure it out quickly. They remind me of a plexiglass shield. You share a bit of your heart or your hurt, and they just look at you. Nothing sinks in. Instead, it bounces back in your face. Don't feel stupid or ashamed. They aren't your people. Feel empowered to let go of particular friendships that aren't willing to practice living in vulnerability, just as you are.

I'm challenging you to live in the truth of who you are. Not just the truths of your accomplishments, but also the truths of what you are ashamed of. When you open this door to what you believe feels and looks like darkness, it is immediately transformed into light. A verse in the bible says, "The truth will set you free."(John 8:32) . When your truth is spoken, there is no space for light and lightness to float on in. You feel lighter, free from the chains that held you down.

And most importantly, you created a safe space for your true people to share with you as well. You become a teacher to others. They become students and then teachers themselves.

Live in "vulnerabilidad," a pretty cool Spanish word that means vulnerability.

Truth 6: Pain Is Pain

Your body was not designed to expend energy to other people on an emotional level to participate and have an internal discussion concerning whose pain is deeper.

Most of us reading these words have all lived long enough to know what pain is. When we are young, we describe pain as a cut, a bruise, a broken bone, or a hangnail that desperately needs a Spiderman band-aid. As we grow and experience our first heartache as a naive seventeen-year-old, we begin to tap into what emotional pain feels like. Making our way into our twenties, those of us who are self-aware enough start to recognize the pain that might begin to manifest due to trauma growing up. And eventually, we find ourselves as full-fledged adults riddled with internal emotional unrest that we either look at in the face or entirely avoid. This only causes more pain on a deeper level. To live is to feel pain, but to embrace pain is to love the entirety of who you are.

So many times, I have had people say, "I shouldn't even be talking about what I'm going through *to you!* You've been through hell and back; my problem is nothing compared to yours." The keyword here is "compared." We have this tendency as humans to compare everything. Our cars, our houses, what college our kids get into, our weight, the list goes on and on. That word is toxic. It goes nowhere good. And in the end, someone is always better, wiser, and has more money than we do. We are conditioned to compare. So it makes sense that people would compare the level of their pain with my fight with cancer. It's natural, but the buck stops there when it comes to one's pain. You cannot measure your pain against the pain of others. It's all pain. And how we process, feel, and respond is different for all of us.

For years, I hid behind the shame of my choices, mainly because I was afraid of what would happen if they were exposed. It was self-inflicting pain that, with every passing day, became a bigger open wound that didn't have a Spiderman band-aid big enough to begin to cover it up. I tried first to ignore the pain and anger, but that didn't work. Next, I tried to tap into it through therapy sessions, which, at the time, didn't last too long. I also tried to create more pain through unhealthy choices, but that just led to bigger caverns of darkness and false escape. Throughout this jungle of emotional turmoil, I was slaying my immune system one cell at a time. I was choosing not to look at my pain as something important enough to become clean with. I expected my physical body to deal with it.

I hated that phrase growing up. When someone said, "Just deal with it," I felt like I had no say. It's an easy out, a kind of end-of-the-story feeling. That's precisely what I said to my body for years and years. "Just deal with it, body. You can handle it. Buck up." Then along came cancer. Cancer of the blood. As Louise L. Hay notes in her book, *You Can Heal Your Pain*. "Blood represents joy." I kept my physical and emotional body in a joyless state for too many years. My blood began to boycott against me since the boss wasn't providing the right working conditions for the job.

Throughout these thoughts and experiences of pain, my conditioned brain said, "Well, at least I'm not going through what this other person is dealing with." When you compare your pain with someone else's, you take away from the importance of your pain. Why do we do that? Why do we feel we aren't important to the most important person in the room? Ourselves! We often forget that words like sadness, grief, fear, disappointment, and hopelessness are just as important as celebratory words like joy, happiness, and love. The irony in this way of thinking is that if we begin to heal the wounds and acknowledge the pain, we open the door to experiencing the freedom that comes with it. This scary and complicated process requires a brave and vulnerable soul.

I never expected my life to be where it is. I recently opened a document in my email where the first two sentences read, "Congratulations, you are officially divorced. See the court documents attached." I had a sinking feeling in my stomach, a mix of anger, sadness, and irritation that the person who wrote this email used the word "congratulations." This wasn't a celebratory moment. This was a sad moment. If I could invent a word bigger than pain, that is the word I felt. But I couldn't find it.

However, the days after reading this email, I began to feel a lightness that I didn't know I could feel. I felt a sense of liberation, freedom, and empowerment. In a roundabout way, my teenage girls thanked me for the difficult step their father and I had made amicably. Joy and happiness are slowly growing. There will be dips where I will do my best to feel it all. Overall, I anticipate the good to continue being good. From there, the good moves toward "better." The better is moving toward peace. When one's pain is recognized without shame, it opens the door to the good, the better, and eventually, peace.

There is a verse in the bible that I've always connected with. "Count it all joy when you fall into various trials, knowing that testing your faith produces patience. But let patience have its perfect work, that you may be perfect and complete, lacking nothing" (James 1:2-4). Can I apply this verse to my divorce? Yes, I can. If you follow Christ and disagree with me, that's okay. I am not manipulating this verse to justify the choice Kyle and I made together. I do not believe Christ wants to see his children unhappy, lonely, and sad. I cling to this verse because joy does abound in its own way after and through moments of discontent and suffering. I am "perfect and complete" in the love I offer myself. I am perfect and complete when I honor and feed every cell in my body with goodness and truth. In addition, we must sit in the valleys of despair, darkness, and tears to anticipate and eventually live freely in the joy to come. Scripture states, "Weeping may endure for a night, but joy comes in the morning" (Psalm 30:5).

You will see others navigating through difficult and painful experiences. It is not your responsibility to compare your pain to theirs. When you do, it diminishes the self-love you are offering to yourself. You can send a note of encouragement, make a meal, or send a thoughtful text. You can also prepare a delicious dinner for yourself. This is not a selfish but a necessary way of thinking. You can give in ways you feel led, but always give yourself more. Always honor where you are in the moment. Every cell in your body depends on you daily to make yourself the most important person in the room. Separate your being from those around you. Your body was not designed to expend energy to other people on an emotional level to participate and have an internal discussion concerning whose pain is deeper. It's your pain. Own it. Sit in it and know that "joy always comes in the morning." Even if you can't anticipate when that morning will be.

August 2022: Purple Poison

I was taken almost immediately in an ambulance to Jersey Shore Medical Center. As I'm wheeled on the gurney into the ambulance, I clutch tightly to my computer bag with my laptop, phone, and wallet stowed inside. I bring my laptop anywhere I know I might be waiting. In this case, I assumed I would be waiting just a few hours in an ER waiting room, as I did a few nights ago.

The ambulance has a black interior and is incredibly sterile. Unlike The Grey's Anatomy ambulances, this one carries nothing: no monitors, oxygen tanks, tubes, or other medical emergency equipment. I stare at the ceiling, and my eyes suddenly start to feel dry, and I realize I'm not blinking. Occasionally, the driver puts on the sirens, and I envision cars pulling to the side, just as I have done hundreds of times. I hear my mother's voice. "Sarah, every time I pull over for an ambulance, I pray for the person inside." This time, that person was her daughter.

There is a flurry of activity as soon as I arrive. I'm set up in an air-purified room separate from the other rooms on the floor. It's quiet and clean, and I have a decent view. I don't remember many of the details of the first two weeks of my admission. Doctors, social workers, dietitians, and hospital chaplains are just a few people who would filter in and out of my room daily. I'm overwhelmed; I smile and nod at everyone, and I don't know what questions to ask because I realize my course of treatment is still being decided.

I feel trapped, taken off guard, and pinned up against a wall. I resented the facial expressions everyone seemed to rehearse before entering my room: professional and kind, yet with glimpses of pity. I could see it in their eyes. I didn't need to see behind their masks. The eyes are the emotional connection centers between two energetic beings. I imagine the conversations at the nurse's station upon my arrival. "Ugh, we have a 44-year-old mother of five coming in with AML. This is the part of my job I don't like." I can hardly believe I'm here. Life feels pretend.

It's the day of my first Chemotherapy treatment, and I'm not sure what to expect. I sit with my legs long under the blankets people have gifted me, staring out the window. I don't know what I feel. I don't feel anything. My sister and mom are in the room with me, settling nervously into the blue vinyl office-type chairs. My sister is quiet, and I know she's processing. My mom makes small talk with me in hopes it will distract me from the event about to take place.

Three nurses come in wearing face shields, latex gloves, and blue surgical gowns. One carries the medicine; the other two are there for administration purposes. Numbers are read between nurses, IDs confirmed, dates confirmed, and a steroid injection is given before the procedure. It burns. I wince and grip the bed rail tightly. My mother starts to sniffle and goes to the bathroom to collect herself. I want to take her pain away; I want to wipe my sister's eyes, which are filling up quickly with tears. They are both mothers. And mothers feel pain deeply.

A friend of mine who fought her own battle with breast cancer said that I shouldn't refer to chemotherapy as just "chemo." It's important to remember the healing part of this word... therapy. The young twenty-something nurse with gleaming blond hair stands on her tiptoes as she hangs a bag that resembles purple Kool-Aid.

Flashes of my 8-year-old self making the summer drink in my mom's plastic pitcher, which was only designated for lemonade, iced tea, or Kool-Aid, come into my mind. I smirked when I recalled always adding extra sugar but being careful not to be caught. They refer to this type of chemotherapy as "Purple Poison." I winced the first time I heard this phrase. I'm jolted inside. Don't I have enough poison in my body as it is? It would be much better for patients to have a softer name for this medicine. I choose instead to refer to it as "The Purple Protector."

The nurses leave, and the room is silent. My mom, sister, and I watched the purple liquid slowly move down the IV tubing. It doesn't feel like a momentous or celebratory moment; it feels more like a moment of somber respect. And then, just like that, the medicine makes its way through the PICC line neatly secured on my upper arm. I breathe out a sigh that contains everything from fear to relief. My body then melts into the bed for the next two hours as if it's surrendering to this blanket of protection that I am confident will work to rid my body of Leukemia. Even if I didn't believe it, I said it out loud enough times that my body wouldn't have a choice. The thought that it wouldn't work didn't even cross my mind.

Up until now, I never knew what chemotherapy looked like. I had no reason to need to know. I didn't want to know. This was possibly an act of avoidance as the word alone was enough to send chills down a spine, similar to when Harry Potter first mentioned: *"He Who-Must-Not-Be-Named, did great things-terrible, yes, but great."* (J.K. Rowling) And now I find myself in this place where I'm forced to come face to face with this thing, this word, this form of poisonous treatment that is supposed to save my life.

The treatment is complete. My mom and sister have left to go home to handle dinner for the sandy and sunburnt 7-year-olds who have spent the day on the beach. I am here in the company of zen-style coloring books, an ocean-themed puzzle, specialty ginger candies, fancy organic body lotions, and plush blankets, all gifted to me. And I'm angry. Just angry. I'm too tired to do anything about the anger, which makes me more furious. I have a disease I didn't ask for, I've submitted to some "purple poison" concoction that's supposed to kill that disease, I'm trusting in strangers I do not know, and everything that happens from this moment on is entirely unpredictable and out of my control.

Being in control is what I do best. Things work when I know how they are going to work. My calendar is taken care of ahead of time, emails are responded to promptly, soccer fees are paid on time, and there's lunch money in school lunch accounts. I take pride in my control tendencies. It's worked for me in the past, except for now.

I look at the window of my hospital room door and notice the shades are closed. I'm thankful. I'm tired of new faces coming in; some of them are there for connection and sympathy, while others are there to do their job of recording vitals and then leave. I want no one, absolutely no one, to walk through that door. I pound my fists into the bed, and the fire within me pours out. I envision ripping out the plastic tubing connected to my port.

I imagine what the staff would do if I were to get dressed in the clothes I wore three days ago, the only clothes I had, and walk out of that hospital. I like how this story unfolds in my mind, but I realize it works better on the big screen. I'm angry at the dumb coloring books and wish I could rip them into a hundred pieces. How is coloring supposed to make me feel better? If anything, it's going to remind me of how sick I am because I haven't colored since I was twelve years old! And why would I want to color now? I don't want to do puzzles of the ocean. I want to be at the ocean. I cry so hard it hurts, and it hurts worse this time because of all the other times. My body is sore from simply crying.

This mini breakdown took place while I was wearing a purple, long-sleeved Athleta shirt given to me by my cousins. I remember this small detail because what follows might be the most life-changing thought or moment I've ever had. The moments in life that deeply impact us emotionally also come with the sensory details of the world around us. If the thought, memory, or circumstance didn't matter emotionally, our brains would have no reason to remember details such as long-sleeved purple shirts. I cross my arms in front of my chest, sink deeper into the thin hospital pillows supporting me, sniffling back the remaining tears, and then it hits me. The words fly at me so quickly and force me to take an inhale that feels larger than what my ribcage can handle. *I chose Leukemia. It didn't choose me.*

I'm sobered, still, frozen, and fixated on the far-away water tower I see through my hospital window. And I'm in awe of this truth. I smile amidst the absurdity of it all. Why the hell would someone choose Leukemia? No one in this game of life would want to chance this wild card if they had a choice. But I chose it, and I knew, in some backward way, that I would be glad I did. Because everything that happened from that exact moment on would change the trajectory of my entire life. My life needed a rebirth. It needed to be turned upside down and poured into a colander. I needed to evaluate why my joy was non-existent, why crying behind cheap sunglasses on the way to the beach with my kids became the norm, and why I

61

always chose to put myself last. If it was going to take 49 days of hospital isolation to learn, I was up for the challenge. My life was on the line here in more ways than an awful diagnosis. I reached for the blue makeup case beside the fancy ginger chews on my bedside table. I pulled out my bronzer as I knew it had a mirror. I held the tiny mirror directly in front of my eyes. And I repeated out loud over and over again, *"You are not going back. You are not going back. You are not going back..."* I felt a chill, knowing this moment would stay with me for the rest of my life. The life that I now have the power to choose, and the life where I would someday say thank you to Leukemia.

The weeks following the purple poison involved waiting, daily blood count checks, limited visitors, loneliness, a confluence of dark emotions, and feeling as though I had no control over anything. Something as simple as taking a shower was difficult, and choosing to stay in bed seemed like the easier option. But staying in bed meant that I would be losing, and cancer would be winning. So I took on these tiny yet huge challenges and embraced them to prove to cancer that I was still in charge.

Cancer was my enemy, and I wasn't giving up until it started to feel like my friend. Push away an enemy, and they will always come back stronger. Quietly embrace them, speak gently, and be forgiving. Eventually, you become friends. You look back at your history and laugh at the disagreements or incidents that caused the division, and you realize you wouldn't be where you are today if it hadn't been for that former enemy.

A few weeks had passed since my first round of treatment, and I knew that the results would be revealed soon. I was nervous but confident. Scared but strangely empowered. The day had arrived. I sat in front of my breakfast tray, which never changed—a banana, cream of wheat, honey, and cranberry juice. Since hospital coffee tastes like shit, my dad lovingly invested in a pink Keurig that technically was not supposed to be part of my room as everything was Dr. approved. I appreciated my dad's gesture and related it to buying me a souvenir on a family trip when I was 8. Something to make me happy momentarily. I didn't care to ask, and I don't think they blamed me for having it there.

I hear the hand sanitizer wall machine outside the room make its usual sound. My nurse is here for a vital check. Instead, the door opens quicker than usual. Dr. R walks in so fast it seems like he's floating. His energy is light, and his poker face is terrible. He holds a few folded-up papers with penciled numbers scratched all over. I've always envied a doctor's handwriting and wondered how pharmacists can read it.

He stands at the end of my bed to ensure direct eye contact. Emotion is read through the eyes, energy is transferred, and an unspoken language is always there if you are willing to listen. His dark, brown, and trusting eyes told me first. His voice was just confirmation. "Sarah, it's gone. The treatment brings you to a complete response." I reply with maybe the dumbest phrase I've said my entire life. "So medicine works?" He laughs, but not at me. He laughs because he knows how deep this diagnosis runs on many levels. And he knows that patients like me question if any medicine has a shot at kicking something as big as Leukemia out of my body. "Sarah, you are cancer-free."

He leaves; I take a breath and sit in this moment for as long as I need. I want no one to know until I've fully embodied it.

The following days involve waiting for blood counts to rise to a point that will allow me to go home safely. My treatment involved destroying my immune system to eliminate cancer and then starting to rebuild. I cling to the hope of every 8 am lab report, hoping I'm on the right track to head home. The numbers fluctuate, and I'm frustrated, but eventually, the Doctors feel as though I'm stable enough to return home.

It's August 28th. A full 49 days from July 11th, when I made my first appearance in the hospital. It was the day I was going home. My favorite nurse made sure that she was the one helping to pack up my room. Hospital staff teased me as I replaced my dull hospital room with a 40 40-something dorm room. Pictures on the wall, motivational signs, a pink Keurig coffee pot, a mini bookshelf, and a diffuser for essential oils. Secretly, they loved coming in because it didn't feel sad and lonely like so many other rooms.

My nurse, Ally, was someone special. She was young enough to be my daughter, yet related to me as her peer, and as if I were the most important person in the room when she was taking care of me. She took extra care with port changes and flushes. She brought me specialty teas from her home kitchen and made sure to put aside the strawberry Ensures in the hospital fridge because she knew I liked them the best, and that was the flavor that went the quickest.

My dad was there to bring me home. He came into my room, and I could tell he was crying. His eyes were puffy, and his smile was that of relief. He was taking me home. But in his mind, he was bringing home his little girl and not his 44-year-old strong businesswoman of a daughter. And I didn't fault him for seeing me that way. I would feel the same if one of my girls were in my position. Children will grow and start their own families, but as parents, we will always see them as little because little is when we feel their love the most. And everyone at every age wants to feel loved.

Ally makes a quick phone call to the nursing station. "We have a bell ringer!" She was smiling, and her gaze was on me the entire time. My dorm room is loaded up and ready to go. My dad carries most of the bags while the rest hang neatly off the wheelchair, which takes me to the bell. Ally wheels me down the corridor, and my dad walks behind. I see the crowd of nurses, aids, and other staff. Smiling, they circle the nurse's station, and I can tell it's genuine. I know I'm not just another bell ringer. I keep them returning to Brennan 2, the Leukemia floor at Jersey Shore Medical Center.

I ring the bell, and I feel silly. It doesn't feel celebratory, so I fake my smile and play the part. Since then, I've had lots of time to reflect on why I felt this way. And I figure it's because this bell thing was never up for debate. It's more for the watchers than the patient. If they find themselves in this position, they will have my story to draw from, giving them the courage to press on. I knew from day one that the bell would ring because there was no option for it not to.

Truth 7: Stop Chasing

The harder we try to steer the ship, the less rest we have between the ebb and flow of waves.

I do not like New York City. I refuse to use the word "hate" because it has always felt vulgar and is overused when it comes to simpler things. Saying words like "hate" embed themselves within you. Your cells respond to the negativity and spur more negative comments and views on life. Using words such as "do not like" is a softer replacement and can still express what you are trying to say.

I've tried several times to like the city. I've done the American Girl Doll thing. The Lego Store thing. The Christmas tree and ice skating thing. The museums, Central Park, Magnolia bakery, and the list goes on. I'm not a native, so my short list of how I've experienced NYC will probably make the locals cringe. I'm sure there are a thousand other parts and hidden places of the city that are exotic and make it special for what it is. I haven't seen those places and likely never will. But I know that even these hidden crevices of the greatest city in the world would not make me like it any better.

I don't have a long list of reasons why I dislike the city. I don't like it because of the movement and the pace. All of these people are going in different directions. AirPods are locked in tight, heads are down, and bodies weave in and out of one another, brushing against each other. The cars are the same. And even though the chaos has a weird beauty, it's the energy I will never connect with. Everyone seems three steps ahead of themselves. They are rushing, moving, striving, and pushing. It reminds me of the classic children's book

Go Dog, Go! By PD Eastman. I liked this book as a child. It has a simple script and an even tone throughout the book. The reader feels at ease seeing pictures of dogs on trees, in houses, in water, and sleeping. And then, the energy and flow of words abruptly change. The dogs rush out of bed and move at full speed in cars. All in a straight line, all following one another. The reader doesn't know where they are going, and it's implied that the dogs don't know either. A tree is far off in the distance. The dogs scurry out of their cars and manically climb a ladder to the top of the tree.

"A dog party, a big dog party!" There's no explanation why there is a dog party; it's just a party that is sweet in its own way. It's busy, there is lots of movement, and each dog does its own thing. One dog is sleeping. That's my favorite dog.

And that's what NYC feels like to me. Everyone is rushing off somewhere. They will likely still carry the same energy that brought them there when they reach their destination. Maybe not physically, but certainly mentally. The harder we try to steer the ship, the less rest we have between the waves.

As humans, we chase. We chase the next promotion. We chase relationships through internet dating sites. We chase money. We chase friendships. We chase the next fad diet. We get so wrapped up in the chasing that the feeling of waiting is lost. We don't like waiting because it feels uncomfortable and challenges us to accept ourselves. And when we sit with who we are, there is self-discovery and often the kind of discovery we don't like. Our chasing covers the messy discoveries we don't want to look at. This chasing might get us where we "think" we need to go, but through this process, we limit what "could" be.

What if we didn't see the tree in the distance? What if we didn't feel pressured to follow the cars in front of us frantically? What if we take a walk and notice what's around us instead? When we practice this type of living, we allow things to come to us. I'm not suggesting complacency. Self-awareness must still be strong enough to create a clear vision and a well-defined destination. However, you can reach that destination with less movement and much greater trust. We are afraid to trust the process of life out of fear. The more you try to control and navigate things, the more it will push back. Life has a plan for you, and it's a good plan. Each action reacts. Each conversation, each interaction, and each decision we make directly correlate to the system of where life could take us and what it wants to take us if we allow it.

Cancer woke me up. The day of my diagnosis, my life stopped and then restarted. I spent hours and hours alone in hospital rooms with time to reflect on how I was living pre-Leukemia. I built a successful business, but was unwilling to hire anyone out of fear. What if they didn't represent my work the way I wanted it? So, I worked myself into a state of sickness. I was living in a loveless marriage for far too long, simply out of fear. If I let go, then what?

On a cellular level, my body realized it was not important enough for it to continue to take care of me. I said "yes" to everyone who needed help. I did this out of fear for the other person. What would happen to them if I did not give of myself? This is a twisted way of thinking because I'm not responsible for them. I put myself aside for others and continued to fuel my illness unknowingly. And there was a high in all of this chasing. There was a financial kickback in my business. There were accolades from the people I helped. There was recognition in the community. Highs were there, but they were minimal. So, I found the next thing to chase—seeking more business opportunities, more hours at the gym, and less yoga. I was chasing health through intense workouts, which ironically made me sicker and not healthier. I was constantly tired, but I took pride in being tired. It was all a lie; it was all ego, and I had nothing to show for it except a self-inflicted road to death.

I refuse to live that life again. I now know the truth. Chasing might bring you to a momentary destination, but ultimately, it's unfulfilling. And very likely, it's not the destination life wants for you. Life wants you to be happy. Life wants to use your gifts, talents, ideas, and passions in this world, but not at the expense of your health.

It took me a life-threatening diagnosis to teach me that my life can be richer when learning to trust the process. And the process is scary as shit. A choice to end a 22-year marriage feels like you're falling out of an airplane. I didn't know where I would land or what the damage would be. A choice to dissolve a thriving business that was a huge part of my identity. The difficult choice of detaching from friendships and people who didn't serve my overall well-being or align with my values.

When we disconnect from what we intuitively know is bad for us, we create space for the unexpected to happen. Again, I am not saying we should sit on the couch and binge on Netflix while scrolling mindlessly through social media, awaiting life's gifts. We can work more authentically in our jobs. Our relationships are richer because we now have space to be present in conversation. Our choices aren't as challenging because we've allowed our inner power to align with the power of life. And those two powers together can produce some pretty excellent opportunities. The harder we try to steer the ship, the less rest we have between the ebb and flow of waves.

Stop striving. Stop chasing. Stop wanting more. Start living "in" your body, rather than letting the world and others dictate what is best for you. Your authentic self knows what you need, but it requires you to be vulnerable and take the scary steps that most others won't take. When you tap into your authentic self, you will attract the energy that matches your own. *Your people* will find you. Your old circle of people might reject you, judge you, and talk about you. This is not about you. It is about them. They can't imagine living a life of healthy risk-taking.

Peeling back the layers of the self-doubters around us is not our work. It's theirs to discover if they are willing. But it's easier for most to follow the crowd in a straight line, going to the same tree, and falling into life's unfulfilling destinations because we haven't let life take us to the mountains that hold the trees.

Truth 8: Nothing's "A Shame"

When left unrecognized, shame is a precursor to the disease of emotional dysregulation.

It's 6:20 in the morning. I stand on my gym's green turf, representing a tiny corner of solace where tears are shed disguised as sweat. It's a Saturday, a morning post, another not-so-great series of decisions the night before. I look at myself in the clever mirrors that make everyone look four pounds lighter. I wonder how much extra money a gym pays to install these mirrors. It is a subtle and wise business decision to keep members coming back. I see bags under my eyes, and I feel bloated and tired. I'm disgusted with myself. *What was I thinking?* I wasn't thinking. I was disconnected from my body and replayed the visions of a night that felt like it meant something at the moment, but just a few hours later, represented a deep shame and self-inflicted judgment.

I am knowledgeable about emotional dysregulation, having studied it for the past few years. I've presented over a hundred workshops on different subtopics, but the irony is that I've never really embodied the core principles of my way of living. Isn't that the way a lot of us live? The cobbler's children who have no shoes philosophy. Mid-kettlebell swing, it hits me. The phrase flies into my brain and presents as neon-colored words on a billboard along a busy highway.

I scramble for my phone to write this gem into my notes:

"When left unrecognized, shame is a precursor to the disease of emotional dysregulation."

When we live in the shame of our choices, we give ourselves zero forgiveness or a sense of "getting out." We get used to the shame and the disgust, and rather than trying to heal from it, we allow it to be a silent monster that eats us from the inside out. It's a part of our identity, so much so that we become accustomed to living in the angst, rather than knowing what it might feel like to be curious about it. And since we become blind to the depth of its destruction, our emotional body begins to disintegrate and, at the same time, acclimate to this toxic way of muddling our way through life. Emotions shift into several gears at once. We can't distinguish between fear and anger, or sadness and disappointment. We confuse happiness with momentary pleasure. Shame is the bully spearheading the mess in our heads. Its fangs are so sharp, and its wit is unmatchable that love, acceptance, forgiveness, and healing find it easier to succumb to its talons versus stand in the truth.

Go to a bar and don't have a drink. And then watch. Notice the interactions between people. Notice all of the similarities these strangers share. They laugh and joke because alcohol provides freedom and a means to lock up the shame behind the doors we don't want to open. Women sit at the bar like wallflowers for their men. Most aren't there for their enjoyment but instead for their availability. I assume that many of these women didn't want to go out at all. She thinks it will make her man happy, or possibly a man she does not know yet. I realize that this is not true for all women. Some sit at the bar in healthy relationships, or are single and confident. But being a woman myself, who had bathed myself in shame for far too long, I justified the bar stool I sat on with a 'why not' attitude. The energy of bar scenes is often characterized by lonely people who want other lonely people to be their friends, even if only for a short time. The next day's headache is an uncomfortable consequence, but it's a small price for avoiding what we don't want to feel.

It needs to be understood that energy attracts like energy. If you like smoking pot, you attract others who do the same thing because you compare notes and have fun doing this together. You are avoiding. If you get sucked into cheating, you attract others who have done the same because it validates the bad decision you know you are making. You are avoiding. If you are an overeater, you might have a restaurant friend who enjoys sampling the All-You-Can-Eat buffets in town.

Using food for momentary pleasure, just like alcohol, to stuff down past trauma. You are avoiding. Eating disorder friends find solace in one another because they get each other. There is no judgment when one removes croutons from a salad and asks for no dressing, cheese, or beans. The greens and the salt on the table are what's left. They are avoiding. If you pride yourself in being a class mom, business owner, soccer coach, school board member, and the mom who sells the most mums for the school team... You are avoiding. In all of these scenarios, there is no time to feel. Because feeling means tasting the bitterness of shame of who you thought you would never become.

Next, watch children play at a park on a sunny Saturday afternoon. This is the opposite of the energy and interactions in a bar scene. These little humans are still close enough to the source and have not had the pains of life silently define who they are on a cellular level.

73

They play with clear minds, they are creative, and most of them are non-discriminating against other children or themselves. They are present. They actively play without expecting a result. They live entirely in the moment and are unknowingly practicing self-love. They live in love through swing sets and the game of chase. They are not hiding behind anything. They are living in unending joy. Their pain comes in physical, felt, and not yet emotionally embedded.

Yet, on the other side, shame begins to feed on parental comments or careless caregivers. It is where shame gains momentum from feeling like needing a math tutor in high school makes them feel stupid, or being diagnosed with ADHD separates them from others. If you are a parent, this is not meant to guilt-trip you into recalling all the possible ways you have damaged your children over the years.

Accept the fact that you have failed, hurt, and disappointed them. And understand that someday your inadequacies will be sifted through with their therapist, and that's okay! Be proud of your 24-year-old who seeks out therapy for the ways you might have screwed them up. Truth is... none of us knows what we're doing in any of the roles we play. Especially parenting.

I grew up in a home where the phrase, "That's such a shame," was a fallback comment for everything from a teen dealing with addiction to a failed marriage. The phrase made me cringe as a child, and it makes me cringe today. Nothing is empowering or positive in this sentence. It's empty and full of judgment. It's a stop-gap for the outsider to practice compassion for the pain the other might feel. Nothing is a shame other than not offering love to those who most need it.

When we are brave enough to forgive ourselves for the choices that make us feel bad, inadequate, and unloved, we open up to all the other emotions. This takes time, but eventually, the gears of love, anger, disgust, fear, and pain move in a beautiful, rhythmic harmony. Detaching from the unhealthy masks of avoidance allows us to create growth and space for healing. This is love in its purest form. Forgiving yourself is love. Sitting and working through unresolved anger toward relatives or friends is a form of love. Being okay with being afraid is love. Giving to yourself in healthy ways is love. Love is the master that tames the beast of shame.

Truth 9: Dauntless

To believe means to put forth and manifest an outcome, and to be brave means to live in manifestation, even if it's uncomfortable.

I love where I live. My town is a small, hardworking fishing town, Friday night football-loving, and as many beach cruisers as there are cars. We are people working hard at regular jobs to provide good running sneakers for budding athletes and modest family vacations. Everyone in town knows each other in some capacity. Friday night football games bring us all together. Kids run with wild abandon under the lights surrounding the field. The bathrooms embody a faint smell of alcohol from the teens who choose to walk the line at a school event. Black and gold are worn with pride, and it is the night where, despite differences, we all share the exact reason for being there: camaraderie, the boys, the school, and the feeling of being a part of something.

But the best time of year in this tiny beach town is summer. As drivers, we don't worry about the other cars around us as much as we are aware of the droves of beach cruisers taking up a third of the road. These kids have it made, and they have no clue. They ride their pastel vehicles with pride and confidence. Some have baskets in the front, others have make-shift milk crate boxes on the back, and others have surfboards hitched to the side of their bike. Those riders move fast. They have one vision in sight. Waves.

I often think of the inlet as our town's heartbeat. A narrow parking lot lines the water's edge. Fishermen are scattered along its edge. People sit in their cars, usually alone, and watch the boats come and go. Big fishing boats roll back to shore with tired, dirty, and strong fishermen working frantically to ensure the vessel stays the course. They decompress at the local bar a few blocks away in a few hours. They stay there for 6 hours before resting and going back out for more. Smaller boats sail out to sea for a day trip. Expensive fishing rods hang off the back, and the captain steers with chest puffed out, feeling great pride in the purchase on which he might struggle to make the monthly payments.

The inlet is a symphony for your sensory system. The boats are all different. They carry their energy and personality. The soothing sound of water, the chirp of seagulls, the smell of diesel, and the salt air represent a small yet powerful fishing town with more power than most realize. Most of us locals take this for granted, and we don't give enough accolades to the brave men and women who dare the uncertainties of the ocean to provide us with branzino, calamari, and swordfish specials at our fancy restaurants.

I sit in my car at the inlet. It's raining, but that doesn't stop the boats. They move slowly in and out of the inlet. I'm crying because it's one of the safest places to cry. People don't see you or hear you. The car offers a cave with a beautiful view.

I cry because my marriage is over. I lean into the steering wheel and grip it tightly. I cry so hard that my stomach aches, and it feels so good. It feels so good because I'm feeling a tiny bit of physical pain that is a drop in the bucket compared to the emotional pain I'm feeling. I'm tired of trying, I'm tired of doing, I'm tired of marriage therapy, I'm tired of fighting, I'm tired of lying to myself, and I'm tired of not feeling loved. I cry because I don't even know what love is. I cry because I can't imagine ever feeling loved. I cry out of feeling helpless, useless, and hopeless. I cry because I feel like my life is defined by cancer. I cry because everything feels unfair. I cry because I never pictured my life to turn out this way.

I lift my mascara-stained cheeks from the steering wheel and see it. I see the words unattached to the massive vessel. I see it as its message. I see it as if God is holding me and giving me a pep talk with one simple word.

The word "Dauntless." There it is in big letters, coming in from its work at sea. This boat is white, with red letters that embody strength and fulfill their role. Someone named this boat, and beneath its beauty lies a story. Maybe the name was given because it takes bravery to head out to sea with waters and conditions unknown. Or maybe whoever named this boat needed an everlasting reminder that being brave is a choice. When we choose "brave," we listen to the voice that propels us forward into unseen waters.

I've never liked the phrase, "be brave." That feels like a demand. Instead, "choose brave." Decide in your mind and take the necessary steps of self-talk to reach a place where you can choose to feel brave and scared simultaneously, brave and lonely, or brave and uncertain about what the action of bravery will bring.

I'm one month into the finality of my divorce. I'm scared as shit, but I'm brave. I'm lonely, but I'm brave. I'm tired, but I'm brave. I'm all the things that scare me into a dark corner at times, but brave is the tiny light that says I can keep pushing forward while honoring the entanglement of emotion within me.

I refuse to return to a life where I chose to lie to myself about being brave. I wasn't brave. I just used the word to cover up my fear, the

78

chaos, and all of the uncertainties from marriage to career and other relationships. I now choose to honor where I am in the present moment. This is true for me. Anything less than the truth damages the cellular orchestra that plays thousands of instruments.

Instead, I will choose bravery to feel a sense of control, rather than having to "be brave." I can choose the brave and also marinate in any other emotion that seems to want to hang out with "brave." I cannot expect the best in life if I'm not brave enough to take chances and expect ridicule.

Be brave with your actions. Your hidden ideas. They are aching for you to notice them. Changing jobs is brave, leaving a marriage is brave, attending an AA meeting is brave, detaching from unhealthy relationships is brave, and doing less and resting more is also a brave act. And you will notice that when you get into the habit of practicing "brave" daily, it becomes fun and addictive.

The universe delights in the individual who takes steps unknown. Because the universe already knows the steps and destination it wants to take you. But the universe needs your permission. It can't do the work for you. There's a verse in the bible that says, "All things work together for good to those who believe." (Romans 8:28) . Replace the word "believe" with "are brave." The writer in me creates a Venn diagram in my mind, overlapping these words to notice how similar they are.

Both have equal outcomes in the destination. To believe means to have faith, and to be brave means to have faith. To believe means to anticipate a different picture of what beauty could look like, and to be brave means to strive toward something unknown and anticipate the beauty that will emerge from it. To believe means to put forth and manifest an outcome, and to be brave means to live in manifestation, even if it's uncomfortable.

A fishing boat sets out to sea with a job to do. Its vision is set on the job, and its goal is to complete and return. It's not a scripted job, and the amount involved is unpredictable. That level of unpredictability is more costly than most. Out in the throes of the sea, a change in wind patterns, a mishap of gear shift in the belly of the ship. All is a chance, yet that ship glides through the inlet with bravery at the bow. It leads with power and shows no sign of weakness. Instead, it believes in the power of God to guide and is willing to adjust as needed.

The captain doesn't ask for directions. The crew works together according to the ship's instructions. The boat will return through the inlet with a story to tell. It will rest, refuel with the best of fuel, be scrubbed, and all things will be put back in perfect order. It will prepare for the next voyage and look forward to the conquest because the previous trips laid the foundation for its confidence.

The bottom line is that you can choose your ship and the body of water you wish to sail on. Many of us choose shiny boats with plenty of amenities. We choose the ones that will receive the "oohs and ahhs" of people along the shore. We choose waters that allow us to see the destination, and we know these waters are safe because many have sailed before us.

I will no longer sail in these ships. Instead, I will voyage in the strong ships and trust that my captain, creator, and God will conquer the unforeseen. I will not burden myself with the pressure of navigating the waters. That's not my job anymore. I will embrace the storms, the calms, and the change in the wind, as these are the things that make one brave in faith. I look forward to the plot twists because they lead to unexpected turns, which in turn lead to endless bounty. Even though I can't define that bounty, I can practice trusting. I can embrace words like "dauntless" in such a way that they become my name, too. *Hello, I've been through a lot of shit in my life, I consider myself Dauntless.*

Truth 10: Break the Cycle

When you begin to break cycles of what is not healthy for you, it is when you start to re-learn and re-birth the "true" you.

My mom did a great job with meals growing up. And I find myself replicating a few of her favorite go-to meals: meatballs and sauce, a beef ziti casserole, lasagna, beef barley soup, and meatloaf. My mom always made meatloaf in a 13x9-inch glass pan. The golden brown meat would come out of the oven, and juices would fill the base of the pan. Fast-forward ten years, and I find myself making meatloaf as a standard meal for my family. Three of my five kids like the meal, which is a win for a large family with varying preferences.

One night, as I mash the meat with my hands, a soothing sensation that reminds me of my Italian grandmother, I glance at the 13x9-inch pan next to me. And out of nowhere, the thought dawns on me. *Why am I using this pan when a loaf pan would better suit the loaf-type shape of the dinner?* I stop the repetitive motion of kneading the meat and smile to myself. I use this pan because my mother did. And she probably used it because her mother did. So I wash my hands, rolling the soap mindlessly longer than usual while thinking about life's patterns. The patterns and cycles we fall into without trying to. I take out the loaf pan, which makes me feel like I'm breaking some family tradition. And I'm super proud of myself for making this little discovery. It's strangely empowering.

Our lives are a puzzle of learned behavior, patterns, and subconscious choices. In many ways, we may find it challenging to take complete ownership of our choices, as most of them stem from the systematic cycles that our cellular self is conditioned to be comfortable with. These cycles and patterns can manifest in various ways, such as through meatloaf pans, or run deeper. They can inform us why we return to abusive relationships—seeking love yet finding comfort in the rejection, as it might replicate a parent who was not emotionally available to us.

Maybe some of us are afraid to be vulnerable, as we were taught that it is more admirable to be strong and tough it out in life. However, that generational cycle of numbed emotions only leads to uncomfortable family holidays at the table because no one is ever brave enough to discuss the "real" issues. And it's not your fault if you fall into this category. Your body and brain don't know how to do this. It's never been modeled.

Everything that you learned as a child was modeled to you and then taught. You learned to walk by watching others; you learned to use a fork with the assistance of an adult, and you learned to talk by listening and practicing. Our learned behaviors when it comes to addiction, relationships, and self-inflicted pain are no different. If we come from the home of an alcoholic parent, it's more likely that we will fall into that category ourselves. This isn't anything new. It's just the truth.

The bottom line is to be aware. And to practice being fully aware. Not partially aware. Being partially aware is allowing yourself to acknowledge the less attractive aspects of yourself for just a tiny bit. Just enough to get uncomfortable. But while dipping your toe in, decide to fall and see them fully. Be mindful of the choices you make and the reasons behind them. If we walk through this life with blinders on, eyes straight ahead, knowing only what we see, we will find that our patterned choices don't always serve our best well-being.

As a child/teen, nothing mattered to me more than horses. I rode them, adored them, drew pictures of them on my trapper keeper binder, and wept heavy tears on October 4, 1989, when the famous racehorse, Secretariat, died. I didn't know the horse and had never met it, but I felt a strange connection that I held closely. All of that to say, I always wondered why racehorses wore blinders. If they wanted to get to the finish line, didn't they have to be aware of their fellow opponents? However, I understood that the reason for blinders was that the jockey was the one directing the steps.

Cycles of addiction and patterns of this life work similarly. Do it a certain way, as you were conditioned to believe. Follow the path that you are taught and modeled to follow. I vote to remove the blinders, try to pass an opponent, and end up falling and twisting an ankle mid-race. This fall, this disappointment changes the cycles of life and how we were conditioned to perform.

Research any famous poet, advocate, author, or change-maker, and you will likely find they come from a life of adversity. This adversity isn't something that chose them. This adversity is something they chose. Why choose the hard path? It's because the easy path is too predictable. Don't link these previous two sentences with cheesy Facebook quotes that insecure people post to look stronger than they are. Choose hard because hard will change you. Making the hard choice is risky. It's not all rainbows and unicorns at the end of difficult decisions, and sometimes you regret making the choice you thought would be good for you.

Not enough people in this world find themselves valuable enough to risk the outcome of what could be the biggest blessing in their lives. I left a marriage. My children got cheated out of a life they wished they had. And yet, I took the risk, as I've found that breaking cycles of unhealthy choices to make myself healthier is one of the most important decisions I've ever made.

I swim through these new waters as a single mom who envisions being loved again someday. As I type these words, I sit beside my vanilla oat milk latte at my favorite local coffee shop. 95% of this book is written from this same spot, sitting on the same wobbly stool tucked away next to the ATM overlooking Arnold Ave., the backbone of a small, Jersey shore town. Today, this latte teased me not to drink it as it might ruin the perfectly shaped white heart the barista carefully prepared. And on this Monday of Valentine's week, serendipity through a frothy drink reminds me that self-love is all that's ever needed.

Choose to love yourself despite the whisperings of others. Break the cycles that carry toxicity and do nothing positive for you. Be curious about what life might have for you if you choose the brave path of change. I've understood what it feels like to walk a tightrope where one wrong blood test or treatment failure could mean tripping into the darkness below. I know more than others how quick this life is and how much more we are worth than we will ever give ourselves credit for.

When you begin to break cycles of what is not healthy for you, it is when you start to re- learn and rebirth the "true" you. You step away from family patterns, lies, and expectations. You figure out who you are as if you are that last piece of a 1000-piece puzzle that everyone fights to fit in. Your body will thank you and celebrate you, and the universe will present opportunities that you could never even imagine scripting in your mind. God wants to give you all that you deserve. But He cannot provide if He is not giving to the unique being He created.

We must thoroughly understand that no one else is getting in our way. The relationships we choose, the jobs we feel stuck in, the unhealthy habits we form, and the return to day-in and day-out routines are all ways we get in our own way. The tighter we feel we need to control, the less space for miracles to happen. Let me say that again... the tighter you hold, the less you receive.

This is not an easy practice. Let go a little, and you will feel less nervous. Let go a little more and feel sad. Let go another step, and anger sets in. Continue to let go until the ache of fear is the only emotion that your body understands. And it's there, on the precipice of falling off that tightrope, that something will happen. Something good. Something unexpected. Something you've been waiting for and seems too good to be true. Why did this happen? It's because you created the space! You are the definer, the author, the illustrator, and the ultimate designer of the following scene change on the stage that you can either choose to dance upon or watch from the nosebleed section of self-doubt.

Truth 11: Say No

Your voice is your most powerful tool for what serves your overall well-being.

I grew up in the days of D.A.R.E. and the "Just Say No" campaign that seemed to have fallen into Nancy Reagan's lap. It was a perfect platform for a first lady to launch, especially since there wasn't much of a curriculum in schools outlining the dangers of drug abuse and addiction. I believe she was genuinely committed to her chosen stance. I'm recalling it and writing about it in the middle of a germ-infested waterpark in Pennsylvania, so it left some impression on me. However, being the cynical, over-thinker kid I was, I wondered if Nike's slogan, "Just Do It," played a quiet role in launching a phrase that would forever have depth behind its meaning. Either way, I've applied the "Just Say No" principle to many things and circumstances, but I learned after my illness that I hadn't used it enough.

For many years, I was the queen of "Yes, I'll do it!" and "Sure, no problem." Responses like "no worries" and "all good" floated out of my mouth without thinking about how I felt. For far too long, I positioned myself as the go-to mom, wife, and entrepreneur, whom many unknowingly took advantage of just because I was there. And I don't blame them! I started to wear my "yessing to death" (almost literally) like a badge of honor. I did this for myself more than anyone else. I'll prove to myself that I can be good, do good, and gain the respect of others.

The plan backfired. Big-time. While trying to be good, I was being harmful to my body. While trying to do good for others, I built silent armies of resentment toward them. My actions were not sincere. They were not honest because I was tired and I didn't want to do good anymore. And as far as the respect from others... that was void. I created an illusion to convince myself that I am important. My striving for accolades made me feel lonelier, taken advantage of, unimportant, and like a doormat. Yet, I kept "yessing" out of fear of what "no" would feel like.

I like the "Just Say No" slogan because it is direct, holds subtle power, and seems accessible to everyone in every situation. The word "just" represents an exact moment. Similar to when a gun fires at the start of a 400m race. It's a moment; it's fleeting, but in this context, it's so powerful. The word "say" represents your power! Your voice, inner truth, and ability to put what you believe you are worthy of receiving into the world. Your voice has the power to tear down or build up. Your voice is the epicenter of your relationship with yourself. Throughout the day, you have conversations with yourself. You second-guess, weigh decisions, and silently curse certain people you are talking to. Your voice is your most powerful tool for what serves your overall well-being. And there's no mistake in why most toddlers' language is centered around the word "no."

Toddlers get a bad rap. Yes, we need to rein in their righteous and self-serving attitudes, too big for their chubby little bodies, but we can also take a step back, watch them, and learn a few things. A toddler waddles around the world and soaks up every facial expression, smell, and piece of nature; the list is endless. They are in a constant state of learning as everything is new to them. While floating through their world of wonder, they encounter an instinctual response that seems to spring from their mouths like a fire sparked from thin air. "No." I don't want to take a nap. "No." I don't want to eat broccoli. "No." I like that toy, not this one. Understand that I'm not giving toddlers the go-ahead to get their way with their world of discovery. I suggest we admire them for their truth-telling without fear of being judged. In the moments of their no-ing, they gain morsels of confidence that will eventually become lost as they grow older.

We live in a world where it should be used more. A boss says to an employee, "I need that article by Monday." The employee has a family trip planned for the weekend. The employee says, "Yes, no problem." The employee now has to say no to quality time with their family because they were too afraid to say, "No, I'll be on a family getaway. I can get the article to you on Wednesday." Your best friend says, "I need to talk to you about something I'm going through. We need to catch up over coffee tonight. My treat." You are tired. It's been a long Wednesday at work. You only want to become one with the couch, melt away into the land of Netflix, and watch a show you have nothing invested in. But instead, you say, "Yes, of course," and almost immediately, you resent your friend. Do you see what just happened here? You said no to yourself! As the most important person in the world, you have just informed your hard-working cells that they must work a little harder because they aren't doing enough.

For many years, I said yes to a marriage that wasn't healthy for me. I said yes to overworking, ensuring that our family's financial security was assured. I said yes to friends who carried emotional baggage that was too heavy for them to talk about, baggage that I thought I could swing over my shoulder to ease their burden. I was numbing and "yessing" myself into an immune system shutdown. The truth is, I don't blame my body for giving up. My physical body tried everything. It tried to keep up with me during a school year in which I gave over 200 presentations to staff and students. This led to a vocal cord nodule, which I needed surgery for. My voice will never be the same again. It kept up with my CrossFit workouts, fitness, and yoga class teaching for years. It kept up with too many glasses of nightly wine during the COVID days. It kept up with me during my short and stupid stint with smoking. It kept up when I chose to stay up until midnight most nights, only to wake up at 4 am for the gym. It kept me going to keep me alive. It kept up with me while I worked 14 hours on Christmas.

My diagnosis was my doing. I ignored the beautiful, intelligent, strong woman hiding under all the "yess-ing" and bad choices. And sometimes I wonder if I kept piling up all this shit so that I could break down and start over. Fake smiles and crying behind sunglasses caused me to ask myself one day while driving to another soccer practice, "What if I just speed up and run head-on into that tree?" I snap out of it and look at my 12-year-old sitting beside me. She looks out the window innocently, AirPods blocking out the world she might be avoiding. I realized at that moment that I'm more tired of living this life, and with death as the option for an out, it might mean that I'm pretty messed up. I never would have acted on those dark thoughts. But the point is that they were there. Hovering in the cob-webbed corners of never saying no and rarely saying yes to the most important and beautiful human being on the planet.

When presented with what doesn't feel right on a cellular level, I "Just Say No." There's no need for explanation and certainly no need to wonder if my saying "no" could inadvertently make someone else's life slightly more uncomfortable. Am I tempted to make unhealthy choices? All. Of. The. Time. It's daily conscious work to practice saying no. And out of all the truths in this book, I would have to cling daily to the fact that *No* is a complete sentence and one of the most healthy gifts you can offer to the most beautiful human being on the planet. Yourself.

Truth 12: Fear Has No Power

The underbelly of fear is void; there is a foundation, but it's filled with cracks, mostly hidden.

If I could get rid of one milk-and-honey motivational quote that people use far too often, it would be this one:

"Face your fears."

People genuinely trying to encourage me during my illness used quotes like these in their cards and through texts. I glanced over them, especially this one. Face my fear of dying? Face my fear of another enormously painful bone marrow biopsy? Face my fear of getting through another lonely and isolated day in the hospital. Face my fear of leaving a marriage and figuring out how to do it alone. Face the fear of returning to my Leukemia doctor every two weeks for 18 months in hopes of positive blood results. My list of "fear-facing" scenarios is endless. Face it? What does that even mean? If I were to create a mental image of the word' fear,' it would look like this. The obstacle or the shitty situation is the fear that stares me in the face. Like David to Goliath, we plant our feet on the ground, waiting for the other to make the first move. Fear is ugly and a coward. It taunts me to join in his mind-fuck circus.

The real question is how we handle fear when we knowingly decide to let it in. Everyone can look at fear from the outside. It's always there, hovering around us like a foul odor, but we have the choice to welcome fear into our world or not. Welcome fear? This might all sound backward to you. But what happens when you welcome what taunts you? If you are smart, you tame it and prove to it that you have control and that it has no power.

There's a knock on the door of my heart, and I know it's not a friendly knock. It's the knock of fear wanting to come in, sweep through, hide in the closet, and create spider webs in the corners of a safe space. I take a breath. I stand straight and tall, all the while pretending confidence over cowardliness.

Well, hello there, Fear, come on in, make yourself comfortable. I'm just going to live my truth and believe that you're just a guest who could take a cue from the phrase "fish and company." What's that? I'm not entertaining you enough? Oh dear, my apologies, but I only entertain guests with something that fills my heart. You have brought nothing to the dinner table of the evening that you expected to have. Go ahead and sulk in the corner and make murmurings about my self-worth. I guarantee that you will run out of sly and empty insults. When you get tired of your pitiful taunting, entertain the idea of sitting on my porch and having a drink. I prefer a rich Merlot in winter and light New Zealand wine in warmer months. I'm guessing you're a bourbon guy? Neat, of course. Let's allow a taste of alcohol to dissolve the wall between us.

I want to be your friend. I want to let you in with the understanding that you are powerless over me. You see, you're no different than those in my life who have taken advantage of me and what I can give them. I've spent my whole life catering to the needs of others for their gain. You are no different. You want something from me. You want an emotional kickback to boost your deflated ego. Fear, let's agree to be friends. After all, I'm not going anywhere, and you will continue to poke my arm like an annoying seven-year-old trying to get what he wants. Honestly, it's just easier to put our fists down and see one another for who we are, separate from any intertwining of

93

thought or emotional dependence. And yes, that Bourbon you're drinking is the finest there is. Only the best for a new friend.

Feed fear with irrational thoughts at 3 am while you can't sleep, and it will grow. Encourage fear with second-guessing and internet searching, and all too soon, you will find yourself living under a daily Eeyore cloud of self-doubt. Like that other milk-and-honey quote states so well,...*What you feed grows* can easily be applied here. Your body has a limited store of emotional reserve until it starts dipping into your cellular physical self. Ever wonder why it's hard to have an appetite when you are afraid? Or the neck pain that tenses over every time that awful thought enters your brain? That's the somatic burden of fear. And trust me, friends, it will destroy you.

I don't believe that we came into this world with a spirit of fear. I think it's learned. A kaleidoscope of memories, family dynamics, parental role models, and, of course, trauma feed the pulse of fear that, if not tamed, will just continue to grow. I've lived my whole life in fear, so I was more comfortable being afraid than being at peace. The adrenaline rush, flushed cheeks, and that heart-sinking feeling all felt like home...over and over and over again. These aren't the pages to get into where this deep-seated fear sprouted from. That's for me to know and for me to understand. Instead, these words are meant to encourage you to see fear, but only if you are willing to recognize that it's a reaction, rather than a mindful response.

I write these words as I sit in the soft leather recliner in a familiar room, awaiting my Leukemia doctor. This appointment is out of the ordinary, as my labs showed a low white blood cell count just a week ago. Ironically, I began this portion of my book about two

94

weeks ago, as I've spent the last seven days practicing what I preach.

The unexpected news of a low white blood cell count sent me into a downward spiral of irrational thought and fabricated lies. I lay awake in the middle of the night and began planning my funeral. I was mentally selecting the pictures Kyle and the kids would add to my memory boards, aligning them with the walls of the funeral home. I pictured police directing traffic outside O'Brien Funeral Home in Brick, NJ.

I felt sad for my kids and my students. I mourned that I wouldn't be able to hold my grandchildren. I decided to write sealed letters to each of my kids, only to be opened on a momentous day, such as the birth of a first child, a wedding day, prom, or graduation. I calculated the money. My head spun out of control in a hundred different ways. Living in the lie that I would not be living had me deciding between an open casket or cremation! I was on a rollercoaster of emotions, flying off the tracks with nowhere to land.

In my conscious brain, I realized this distorted way of thinking couldn't be true. And as awful as these thoughts felt, they also felt safe at the same time. They felt at home. I didn't know how not to be afraid, and it was easier to sink into dark scenarios of death than picture the opposite side of the coin, which could be shiny, long-lasting, and beautiful. And why is that? Why do some of us find a friend in despair, rather than being besties with joy and hope? The only thing I can come up with is that it's hard work to speak against the demons in our brains that whisper false hopes, reinforce insecurities, and encourage self-loathing.

I don't have a doctorate in behavioral health. I'm not a social worker or psychologist, but I am human. And I'm a human who challenges myself to be curious about the hard things. And sometimes, we don't need data and studies to find the answers to why the brain reacts in a certain way. Instead, we need to be honest with ourselves and face our fear, let it in, become friends with it, and realize that it's harmless, like one of those bullies on the playground in third grade who only bullied because they didn't know how to connect otherwise. The underbelly of fear is void; there is a foundation, but it's filled with cracks, mostly hidden.

In the end, my white blood cell count returned to normal. My doctors rolled their eyes at me, laughed, and thanked me for inviting them to my pretend funeral. Fear will become your God if you allow it. It craves emotional weakness, much like Audrey II craves blood in *Little Shop of Horrors*. Don't become Fear's Seymour. You will slowly begin to die on a cellular level from the inside out. And don't just face fear. Even there, you are giving it power. Let it in, become friends with fear, and understand that your new friend is just an insecure bully who doesn't want to be the last one picked for a third-grade recess kickball game.

September 2022: Balancing Act

I am home, and the only thing I want to do is be outside. Forty-nine days of hospital isolation had taken away fresh air, the sound of airplanes and cars, the smell of salty air, and the penetration of sunlight. My senses are heightened, and everything feels too loud, bright, and disturbing. The soles of my feet begin to ache after a couple of days, and I realize it's because they aren't used to walking. My eyes take a while to get used to sunlight, and sitting on the couch at night while watching Netflix feels like a luxury.

The days to follow bring my old life into light. There's so much activity. Everything is moving too quickly. Kids going to the beach, teens running late to work, soccer practices, and all the other life "stuff" that soaks between the cracks. School starts, and my friends help with back-to-school shopping for my older girls. A neighbor brings my younger children to buy school supplies. My oldest has already left for college after saying goodbye to me in my hospital room. This room is just four floors above the room where we first met on the maternity floor of Jersey Shore Medical Center. Life feels too busy, and I don't know where I fit into this chaos.

I'm out of practice, and I try to be patient with myself and, at the same time, thankful for the help of my parents, in-laws, school community, and friends. *How do I start to be a mom again? Are my kids scarred from not seeing me in so long? Do they even care?* These are questions that I can work through if I sit with them long enough. The looming question, the one that grips my chest with a subtle tightness I can't shake, is whether or not my doctors will find me a bone marrow donor. I am relieved that the Leukemia is gone, the treatment worked, the isolation was necessary for recovery, and I have come out relatively healthy. But in my case, the word "healthy" is unsteady. It doesn't carry the same weight as it would for someone else who is cured of a life-threatening disease.

The Leukemia will come back. At some point, it will come back. My bone marrow, the life-generating part of my body, is still not whole. It needs a replacement; unfortunately, there is no available spare yet. My siblings are adopted and, therefore, not a match. My parents have aged out, which has led me to hope that my future may rest in a database of 35 million potential donors.

I am home from my 49-day hospital stay for seven days before I meet with my bone marrow Doctor. We have not met yet, but I like her already. I grieve a bit knowing that my Leukemia doctor will not be as close to my case now that I've graduated to bone marrow land. I brought a trusted nurse friend to my initial consultation with my bone marrow doctor. I needed an extra set of ears that wasn't clouded by emotion and could disengage when the content became too overwhelming. I knew I could count on her for precise note-taking and medical-like questions.

I walk into "Hope Tower" for the first time. I've passed this building hundreds of times during the past 20 years of living on the Jersey Shore. And every time I see the word "Hope," I am inspired by not only the word but the brave humans who walk in every day. It's not the "Healing" or "Life" tower. The building is founded upon hope. Hope for a bone marrow donor, no more treatments, clear scans, remission, and ultimately, hope for life. And here I am. I park illegally in the Walgreens parking lot just a few blocks from the tower. The parking garage is packed, and I don't want to deal with the hassle of driving in circles for a spot and waiting for elevators. I'll take the chance of a ticket. A mindset shift newly informed by cancer. It's the "why not break the rules and see what happens?" So far, my track record is pristine. Not one ticket in 10 months. It's strangely empowering to claim the same spot every visit. I feel like a faculty member at a college with a designated parking space. I wonder if other patients take advantage of this secret, or if I'm the only one who's clever. Cancer will not define the rules, even if the rules come down to where I should be parking.

I wait patiently in the sterile room of the bone marrow transplant floor. My nurse friend is next to me, holding a blue pen and a blank, lined piece of paper, ready to take notes. I'm thankful for her, yet I'm unsettled by her quiet spirit. Upon reflection, I realize she understands the gravity of my situation. She's accompanying her friend to a bone marrow appointment, during which I may or may not have a chance to get a match. And ultimately, an opportunity to continue life.

My legs are crossed, and I gaze at my black flip-flops. The identical flip-flops I wore when I walked into an ER 8 weeks ago with a nagging fever and pain in my side. I am then rushed in an ambulance from one hospital to another to treat my disease better. During the hustle and bustle, I had left one of my black flip-flops at the first hospital. My Oncology doctor returned it a few days later and referred to me as his "Cinderella Patient." I immediately felt a warm and comforting connection as he made me feel human, not just a person with cancer. He made me feel safe. I liked the parallel message as Cinderella eventually escaped her prison.

My foot twitches nervously, and I can't stop. It's comforting and helps settle the anticipation. We are both quiet. We wait, we wonder, and we know my life is still a tightrope of indecision and "what if" scenarios. I don't ask my nurse friend questions about the process because I don't want to know the answers.

My doctor enters the room with a grace that only comes with practicing this role hundreds of times. She is nothing like I pictured. She's petite, slight, and quiet. She reminds me of a grade school friend whose nose was always in a book and was quickly coined as the class brainiac. I imagine her as a medical school student. The one who studied until early morning hours, the one who kept her sights secure and focused, and her heart driven to save as many lives as she could. She wore a mask that hid her smile, but her gentle eyes made up for it. She shook my hand, and that hand reminded me of my mother—soft skin, knuckles visible, and petite.

She sat down casually as if we were two friends out for coffee. She put her notepad aside and leaned forward. She asked about my personal life. She asked what I do, the age of my children, and where I was emotionally. I tried to connect, but I put up my guard as I always do. I wondered if she cared or if this was all part of her interpersonal patient-related training in medical school. I catch myself thinking this and actively push aside my judgments. This is no time to shield feelings with pride. This is a time to be soft, humble, and accepting of this brilliant woman whose job and passion is to save the life of a mother of five fighting for her life.

The appointment ends with hopeful news that a few donors are potential matches. Nothing is concrete. I take note of the doctor's careful choice of words as she explains the lengthy process of locating the donor and trusting the donor will comply with the steps involved in donation. I accept this response as if I had found the golden ticket, just as Charlie had in Willy Wonka and the Chocolate Factory. My favorite part of the movie is when Grandpa gets up from his bedridden state and dances with Charlie around the room after discovering the ticket. I felt like Grandpa. Suddenly alive and happy and well, all the while knowing I'm still "in bed" and the joy of hope might only last so long. I leave the hospital feeling light and celebratory. Upon reflection, I find it ironic that nothing was secure. It was all a presumption on my part. It was as if I pretended that hope was definite and, therefore, I would be okay. I'm thankful for my mind's intuitive response. I was protecting myself without even realizing it.

My parking spot tactic is one I continue to be proud of as I visit Hope Tower three times per week. The process is always the same. I chat with the intake receptionist, whom I'd come to adore. She's motherly and kind and always lets me know how pretty I look. I stay for bloodwork before it is determined whether I need a blood or platelet transfusion. I've become an expert with the numbers. I know what's borderline and stable, and I can now predict what the doctor will order. For the first time in my life, I feel in charge of my health, even though it took a life-threatening disease to make me feel confident in that.

The transfusion area of the hospital holds an energy that I've never embodied before. The nurse calls me back. It's always the same one. He wears burgundy scrubs, knows me by name, smiles, and welcomes me as if I'm walking onto a cruise ship. Instead, I walk to the scale for a weight check and then to the vitals station. I like him. I'm just part of his routine, but he does his best to make me feel as if

I'm not just another number in the line of cancer patients. Eventually, the day for a platelet or blood transfusion is determined. Either way, I'm prepared for the three-hour stay. I don't mind it. My laptop is along for the ride, snacks and coffee are provided, and if I'm lucky, I am set up in a corner suite, nestled away from the many treatment chairs packed close together. I scan the room and know what to expect. Patients wear emotionless stares with a loved one by their side. They tune out to the mindless TV channel before they go to sleep. They are tired, feel cheated out of life, feel weak, and wonder if any of this is worth it. I can't let their actions define my own. I have to rise above what I see. I have to stay positive. I have to fake it even if I don't feel it.

I busy myself by working on invoices for various schools related to my business. I pretend I'm in an office doing very important work. Instead, I'm on a cancer floor receiving blood from some random stranger who spent his lunch break giving blood because he felt a bit guilted into it by his coworker. And I do this alone. Always alone.

September feels like that new pencil smell combined with freshly cut grass. My younger kids are smiling at the bus stop, while the teens half-smile in front of the door for picture documentation, clearly irritated by my need to capture the moment. I'm a little too excited to be here for it all, and I'm allowed to be. I sail through September and act as if everything is normal. I've always believed that if the odds are against you, one of the cures is to "fake till ya make it." I push aside the "hope" for a donor and pretend I'm living life pre-Leukemia. I find myself wandering through Kohl's Department Store just because I can. I spend 45 minutes of my day walking the boards of the Jersey Shore. September is bliss here, but only the locals know about this yearly secret.

I take myself to lunch alone and admire the people around me with normal functioning bone marrow. I clean out closets, donate to Goodwill, and nap daily. I am aware of the necessity of being gentle with myself. And I realize how sweet this life is for the very first time in my life. The tiny moments when my children hug me on their own. Waiting in line at the Starbucks drive-through while listening to Johnny Cash. I plan a nice dinner for my family and then take the time to prepare it. A meal tastes better when love and attention to detail are in check. All of the meals tasted good through September.

I will be the first to admit that pre-cancer, I was never a good board-game mom or going-to-the-park mom. I got impatient and wasn't a huge fan of pushing swings or assisting with monkey bars. The inviting benches in the shade under trees seemed to be there for decoration as they taunted me with the "possibility" that I might be able to sit down. The other moms were huddled in clusters throughout the playground. I had three categories for the park moms. There were the *First Baby* moms. They were the ones who compared labor stories, prided themselves on fancy diaper bags, and proudly declared how helpful their husbands were with night feedings.

Then there were the *Fitness* moms. They usually didn't arrive until 10 am as they attended their 8 am gym class. Their toddlers were cranky from being in gym daycare for an hour, and they exuded pretend confidence as they sported their fancy leggings and crop tops. Most of them felt good about themselves, but hid their frustrations and life problems well. *First Baby* moms watched them with envy, wanting to be like them someday.

And then there were the *Old* moms. Those in their late 30s or early 40s, with three or four kids in tow. These moms looked at the younger generations and didn't envy them. Instead, they were well aware that someday the blushed-face beauties would be tired, possibly divorced, and ache for the days when they only had one child. I stayed away from all of the moms. I learned early on in my parenting that very few felt the need to highlight their child in every sentence. I also learned to keep my circle small and only let others in who were vulnerable enough to be honest about how hard this parenting thing was. Those were my people. The moms who had nothing planned for dinner, scraped their diaper bags for the snacks they had forgotten to bring, and asked how I was doing. Those were a few. I often found myself alone at parks.

I mindlessly push swings and watch the clock, forcing myself to stay 45 minutes. We visited lots of parks. I've always tried to get my kids outside as much as possible. Parks, boardwalks, beaches, orchards, and snowstorms. But it all takes work, and many times, I resented the laborious task of zipping up snowsuits and finding a missing glove so they could play in the snow for just 11 minutes. I felt guilty when I wasn't present with my kids, as I had given up an excellent teaching job years ago to be home with them. I'm sure they sometimes felt the obligation when I practiced the "fake it till ya make it" mentality while at parks and playing board games.

It was a gorgeous Saturday morning in September. I wanted to get my 7-year-old twins outside. And on this Saturday, I wanted to go to a park. After 49 days of hospital isolation, I was craving this simple experience that I had once loathed. I picked up a few friends for the twins, and we took a 30-minute drive to a park a friend had told me was worth visiting. The girls sing Harry Styles songs aloud, and the boys discuss soccer while tuning out the girls' off-key verses.

We arrived at the park, and it was huge. The kids bolt out of the car, leaving me to carry four water bottles. They laugh, run, and explore the obstacles. They find an open field nearby. They run without a well-organized plan. One of them yells to me about a trail that had been discovered. We all walk the trails, participate in obstacle courses, and visit a nature center. Eventually, they start to get tired and ask for snacks. I looked at the time and noticed we'd been here for two hours!

I realized for the first time in my motherhood journey that I was fully present with my kids. My body knew of this gift—the sun, the picnic tables, the scraped knees, and the laughing. I was a great park mom that day. It was great because cancer informed me that the simplest of moments can be the greatest memories. Disney World and a trip to Atlantis might not be on the agenda...ever. But my newly invented mindset can make a trip to Walmart with my kids something not to take for granted.

September comes in with excitement, fresh air, and alone time while the kids are at school. I enjoy each day and relish fresh sheets, open windows, and the freedom to go outside. However, a looming and nagging feeling often haunts me, mostly at night, when I'm trying to fall asleep. *What if the doctors don't find a donor match for me? How many months do I have? Am I scared to die? Do I believe in the faith I've been soaked in my entire life? Will I go to hell for questioning that thought?* These thoughts are rational and irrational all at the same time. They collide and never produce a firm answer. I keep this all to myself because no one can relate to the emotional

105

hell these past few months have been. People try their hardest to relate and offer comfort. I take their words, cards, donations, and meals with honest gratitude. I am loved, and I know that. But I get so angry because I still feel alone. And maybe that's what Leukemia wants you to feel. Maybe it's all about the blessing in disguise. To be forced to feel alone, but with your strength. I continue to tell myself that, in the end, this will all be worth it. But will it? And what does my end look like?

Kyle and I continue to move through the motions of daily living. We are still separated, and that works best. I know these past few months have been hard on him, and I understand that he can't process this disease emotionally on a deeper level. He escapes in ways that bring temporary enjoyment, and I get that. I try not to shame him for this. I understand the need to escape, but I get resentful that I'm the one who gets the short end of the stick. I want to escape. I don't want to be here. I don't want to be the person everyone is worried about. I want to be the person organizing meal trains and finding ways to provide emotional support.

My marriage is over. We both know that. But we are self-aware enough to understand that nothing can be done until this storm is behind us. We are good parents. We screw up and make massive mistakes. Who doesn't? Everyone takes on this parenting role and navigates each wave as it comes. Some waves you float over, and others knock you on your ass, where all you can do is try to come up and get your bearings. And when the water is calm, the next set of waves comes along.

Kyle will forever be one of my best friends. I'm sure of this. But when it comes to a marriage, best friends don't cut it. Something has always been missing, and it's taken a life-threatening disease for me to feel brave enough to do something about it. I'm worthy of love. Real love. A love that will stave off the disease that almost killed me.

Truth 13: Your Circumstances Do Not Define You

If you give a negative situation any ounce of power, you might have given it all of you.

I've said from day one of my diagnosis that cancer would not define me, would not have ownership over me, and had no right to sneak its way into my bloodstream and, more importantly, into the life of my immediate and extended family. Even though my body was soaked deep in "blast cells" that were multiplying with every passing minute, I refused to give cancer any more space than it had already taken up in my body. Reminders of its presence were tattooed all over my body. My once-healthy skin tone was now a canvas of disease—the bruises on my thighs, chest, and back. The red, blotchy, acne-like patches on my face reminded me that I was fighting something I had dared to let feel bigger than I could handle.

I couldn't believe I was in this position, but I accepted it. What was the other option? A cowering 44-year-old mother of five sobbing her eyes out in the dark, sterile hospital room, refusing to eat or interact with people on text? Nope. That's not me. I accepted the reality of my situation and trusted the words of a close friend. "You're in the place you need to be. These people know what they are dealing with. Trust them." So I did.

Here's the thing. If you give a negative situation any ounce of power, you might as well have given it all of you. Your circumstances, whatever they are, do not define you. Let me say that again. Your circumstances do not define you! It's essential to recognize that they are a part of you, as ignorance can create a significant amount of emotional unrest. What we avoid always has a way of reminding us it's there. Just lying there beneath the surface of fake smiles and "Yes, I'm great" attitudes that fuel your adverse circumstances to gain more and more power.

And understand that this is way easier said than done. If there were a medal for the best avoider in my thirties and early forties, I would have sheepishly stood on the podium of shame to show off my win. I no longer play that game. It can play me as much as it wants, but I refuse to allow those circumstances to take up much room in my brain. If these thoughts occupy space in my brain, they most certainly make their way to the more complex parts of my body on a cellular level.

I'm a divorced mother of five and come from a highly faith-filled and conservative upbringing. My steps through divorce were daily work against shame and doubt. I vacillated between the inner voices of "You're a fraud, a bad Christian, and a shame of a mother" and "You know what's healthiest for you." Allowing my upbringing to define me and allowing myself to melt into life's big failure as a mom did nothing good for me. Attending church as a divorced mother could be powerful or condemning. I chose God's grace and melted into his everlasting love. Can we all agree that Christ walked among the people, and while He did, He breathed love into every interaction He made along the way? I never questioned my faith. I knew the God I served. I knew He loved me, no matter what circumstances the world might deem shameful and wrong.

Some might read this and think I'm contriving ideas to cover up my guilt and justify my choice. And yes. It was my choice. I left a marriage. I made the choice and will forever take full ownership of the choice, only giving my power to serve positive feedback. And yes, I struggle with the divorced woman role. I grieve what I thought I would have had. I grieve for my kids and what they thought they would have had. No divorce is ever fair to little hearts. They will always be partially broken because of my choice, but then I wonder if my decision to stay would have caused even greater damage. They saw and felt my heaviness for so many years. What was I modeling to my daughters? I was allowing them to see a woman in a marriage who was sad and resentful and stayed there because that's what good Christian girls do.

I'm raising strong girls who will someday realize that part of their strength comes from a mother who refused to allow a life of sadness to define her. I hope they will remember a mom who made the hardest choice of her life to better her well-being. And in the end, I want my girls to understand that they are the most valuable and beautiful gifts on the planet and that they will never settle for anything less than a bouquet of roses, not just on Valentine's Day, but on the "Just Because I love you days." I want what I never had for them. And, like my middle daughter confessed to me one day out of the blue... "I wish you and Dad had split sooner, Mom." Me too, baby girl, me too.

Stop giving things that don't serve you empty power. Be bold and share the hard. Let others talk, mock you, and judge you. Ultimately, your circumstances and where you are have nothing to do with them. It has to do with your growth. Instead, own your mistakes and confess to them for what they are. This is human friends. This is real. This is what many people are afraid to do, fearing what others might think. I can bet you in more ways than one that those who judge only judge because they couldn't imagine taking this reflective microscope on their life. People avoid it; they lack curiosity. People sit at a bar and drink their sorrows away instead of screaming into a pillow. People have affairs to numb the loneliness. People stay in jobs they hate out of fear. People buy houses and boats they can't afford to fill the void that gets deeper and deeper with every swipe of an American Express Card. I used to be one of those people. Mindless and damaging self-inflicting choices were killing me from the inside out. I avoided even glancing at the things begging to have a conversation with me. Leukemia brought me to my knees and shattered me into a million pieces, and it was here I whispered, "Hello, pain, be my friend."

I recently made a final visit to my childhood home of 40 years. My parents made the brave decision to sell a significant portion of our beautiful farm property. It was Easter weekend, and it seemed appropriate to say my final goodbye. I took time to scan as much of the property as possible so that my little girl, teenage, and early twenty-something brain could process the flood of good and bad memories that flowed like intersecting rivers with every footstep.

We attended the Easter Sunday Church service, and it was sweet to see our entire church row filled with our family. My parents were proud, happy, and content. I pictured myself feeling the same way someday, in the hope that my grandchildren would find their way to create a similar memory. I've been to enough Easter Sunday services to know the introductory sermon. It's usually a milk and honey message and a safe one, as the pastor knows he needs to be sensitive to guests and out-of-town visitors. But this service was drier than most. The music was slow and dull. People sang the songs but with little emotion. "Amens" and "He is risen indeed" phrases were voiced at appropriate times, and the hour-long service fulfilled the script outlined by the worship team and pastor.

All in all, it felt like an obligation, not a service, where I was challenged to embody the fullness of Christ's sacrifice for my unhealthy choices. And then I see it. It's like a trailer for an upcoming blockbuster. My brain sees it all playing out on the stage before me. I confidently imagine walking down the aisle and making my way to the podium, where the pastor stands. I asked him gently and with respect if he would allow me to take the microphone. He steps aside, hands me the microphone, and I take a deep breath. My presenter instinct kicks in. I read the crowd, the body language, and eye contact. I figure out what I'm dealing with in a few seconds. And I go for it anyway.

"Hi, friends. I know you have no idea who I am, but I'm asking you to trust me for the next few minutes. We can all agree that today, we celebrate Christ's resurrection, right? This is the day we embody His fullness and power, walking alongside us every moment of our day. It is the day we remember and celebrate his unending forgiveness for our sins. So let's talk about it. Let's talk about the sin. Can we all be transparent and connect with what we hide right now? All of you have things you are struggling with. Maybe you are gambling late at night without your spouse knowing. Or are you drinking while working just to get through the day, and now it's becoming more frequent? Do you look forward to a weekly rendezvous with your colleague? Maybe you're reconnecting with an old high school

crush on Facebook, which feels exhilarating. Anyone stealing small amounts of money here and there from unsuspecting clients? Who wants to talk about it? Who wants to come up on stage and share your hard? Who wants to share the real you?

Understand, I'm not asking you to "confess" as much as I'm asking you to be honest. If we share what most frightens us, it's more likely that others will feel safe sharing their fears. And it's in these moments of unashamed honesty that we can begin to see each other as the fallen humans that we are. Here, we can connect with Christ's forgiveness and feel Him on a personal and cellular level. He loves you! He wants to stand beside you and put His arm around you. He wants you to melt into his non-judgmental forgiveness and bask in his unending love."

I pause my monologue and scan the crowd. Some heads are down and avoidant. I get this. Others have their arms crossed in defense. I get that, too. But there are a few who look directly at me. Their cheeks are flushed; we call this the Holy Spirit's prompting in Christian culture. Whatever it is, these are my people. And they come up, one at a time. Each one shares something they are ashamed of. I celebrate them, hug them, and tell them they are loved —the mood of the church changes. The pastor doesn't ask for the microphone back. He lets me roll with it. The worship team starts to play —the entire 8-minute vision is off-script, and as the Christians say, "God- breathed."

Friends, listen. You're going to screw up. You're going to make mistakes. You will wonder how most of these mistakes even happened. But the bottom line is that these fuck-ups do not define you. You are not the sum of your choices, your life is not permanently screwed up, and you are not a walking disgrace among people. And if they make you feel that way, trust me, they are not your people. Walk on the other side of the street and tell them you are there if they want to walk with you. But it's on this path that you walk among rocks instead of the smoother path that has held space for millions of footsteps, which are too tired to do the walk that requires the work.

Truth 14: If You Feel It, Do It

The whispers require quiet listening and often feel so far off that you can't imagine even stepping on the first stone that could lead you to a destination you know you are worthy of, but are too scared to believe.

I've always thought that some of the most brilliant people in the world are singer/songwriters. Music and words together. Not just music and not just words, but two powerful forces blended. And when this is done well, magic happens. I consider myself a writer, as it's always something I've loved, but to ask me to put words to a song is beyond my reach. Far beyond my reach. So I've admired the greats who can do this so well, and I gravitate toward the old-timers. Johnny Cash is one of my favorites because he was willing to be vulnerable and sing about it. He made despair sound beautiful and rode the wings of hope through lyrics, trusting that maybe through the process, he might find answers for his own life. However, during an interview, I will always return to the infamous quote of the great David Bowie.

"If you feel safe in the area you're working in, you're not working in the right area. Always go a little further into the water than you feel you're capable of being in. Go a little bit out of your depth. And when you don't feel that your feet aren't quite touching the bottom, you're just about in the right place to do something exciting."

Like most things that strike me on an emotional level, I end up creating a mental image in my mind. There I am, walking slowly into the ocean, with no waves, just still. I'm a little afraid, as I've never fully trusted the sea, and I don't think anyone should. She's beautiful, mighty, and gentle, yet makes her superiority known with every ripple. I feel the deep sand in my toes, water crawling slowly up my waist, chest, and neck. I step cautiously forward, and there it is—the drop. One step further, I slip into trusting or not trusting what's there to suspend me. It's in this millisecond of awareness that Mr. Bowie is referring to.

The decision to leave a 22-year marriage.

Gasp.

Could I do it?

Write a book and lay it all on the line for the world to judge.

Gasp.

Could I do it?

Could I stare cancer in the face?

Gasp.

Could I do it?

Letting go of a business I loved dearly and changing career paths.

Gasp.

Could I do it?

And Mr. Bowie has it right. It's that simple. Feel the fear, sink into the increased heartbeats, and doubts that flood like wildfire. And we find as humans that it's easier to take part in the chaos and distress than to bravely make the choices that might be the best redirection of our lives.

So many of us are so far from our true selves that we don't even know who we see when we look in the mirror. We can see the apparent titles, such as mother, father, accountant, grandparent, teacher, and so on. But we can't know the power beneath the surface because it requires us to feel it first. And to feel something that big can be scary. Big means potential, and potential means success; few of us feel worthy of this life.

Scripture states, "Start children off on the way they should go, and even when they are old, they will not turn from it" (Proverbs 22:6). Growing up in a rule-based, black-and-white home, I grew to understand that this verse meant to keep children following the rules, staying in a box, focused on right from wrong, never deviating, and not seeing mistakes as an opportunity for growth. But with time, and after years of parenting under my belt, which I confess I've failed miserably at times—ask my kids.

I now read this verse in a completely different context. If I had a magic pen to re-write this golden nugget of scripture, my version of this verse would say, "Start children off to recognize their uniqueness, talents, and gifts, and don't stop supporting them because one day they will be something great and will feel the fullness of their true selves."

For the past 25 years, my work has primarily centered around working with children. From kids' and teen yoga classes, to grade school teachers and presenters, I've noticed that as I span the development of children, the younger they are, the more they

117

understand who they are. Ask a five-year-old what they want to do, and they will eagerly tell you not just one thing but a list of things that light them up. Ask a 17-year-old; likely, they will not have the answers as quickly. Either they don't care and feel disinterested, don't know, or they are overthinking. The further we grow from the source, the womb, the further we detach from who we are meant to be. And when you multiply this pattern through years of human development, we find ourselves in jobs we don't like, tolerable relationships, and daily routines that replicate Bill Murray's Groundhog Day.

But I can promise you that throughout these adulting years, hushed whispers are brewing beneath the surface of who you don't know you are yet. These whispers are powerful but quiet because they don't want to scare you. They encourage you to consider making life-changing choices that will enhance your well-being. The whispers require quiet listening and often feel so far off that you can't imagine even stepping on the first stone that could lead you to a destination you know you are worthy of, but are too scared to believe.

Start believing that you are separate from every person who walks beside you. There will always be someone better than you at something, but your uniqueness can make your gift and your dream possible. When children don't want to try a new food, the standard adulting phrase is, "Well, you don't know if you like it unless you try." The same rule applies here.

The beautiful part of all this is that all you have to do is create space in your brain and be open to the change, the new beginning, or the dream you want to reach. There's no need to act right away. Dreams and significant changes begin with altering the brain's thought processes. It took me 8 years to muster up the courage to write this book. As I type here in my favorite coffee shop in downtown Point Pleasant, NJ, with 12 minutes to spare before I have to greet 16 5-year-olds for a day of kindergarten, I still don't know if any of these words will matter. But I've allowed myself to sink into the waters unknown that Mr. Bowie is referring to. Putting my wild and, at times, unruly thoughts on paper feels vulnerable and scary. But I'm here with my oat milk and vanilla latte, trusting the process of where this could go. And as sad as it was to leave a 22-year marriage and watch my kids navigate their new life, it's also the bravest thing I've done and has been life's natural medicine to keep my cells full of life and hope.

Regarding life, standing on the sidelines and watching makes no sense. That's the easy way. And that's the way that lots of people take. Emotional work is hard. It's energy; it's exhausting. It's self-reflective to the point where you might discover that who you are is someone you don't want to be. And even if that is the case, it's a great place to be! You've made the discovery.

Step in, dive in, and marinate in the potential of who you could be if you challenge yourself to respond to the calling inside of you that wants nothing more than to change you. And to change means to grow. And to grow means to live more fully. This is an unending process. There is no final destination. It is just continual growth. And in time, you start to feel safe in the waters that once frightened you. And you feel safe because you have learned how to navigate them independently. You are in charge. You are the master with the idea, the song, or the script that lights the way forward. There is nothing braver than standing on the edge with confidence and grace.

119

Truth 15: Cry, Punch, and Throw Shit

But trying to be good only weakened me physically because I was choosing to look past my body's simple need to accept and affirm where it was at.

I'm almost two years post my diagnosis, and I still wish there was a more justified word than anger for the endless hoops of fire I had to jump through. The hoops are less heated these days, but they are still there. Monthly visits to my doctor, with fingers crossed and silencing the lies that my white blood count won't drop below 3.0, is probably the most prevalent thing these days. Other hoops involve awkward stages of hair growth, filling my weekly medicine box, scanning my legs and arms for any unsuspected bruising, and hoping there's no blood when I rinse my mouth after brushing. Subtle signs of Leukemia returning. And anger precedes when I sift through the colander of unrest, while all other emotions trail behind. And since we know that anger results from fear, this all makes sense.

It took me a few months to settle into the fires of anger, but once I did, I didn't know how to stop them. I didn't have to fuel them; they grew independently. Over time, I said hello to anger, became its friend, and navigated life around its taunting. I still feel the stubborn embers burning deep in my belly, and the vision hits me, over and over and over again.

I'm somewhere in the woods, and I'm alone. It's silent. The day is misty, calm, and gray. I fall to my knees beside a stack of 49 white, dollar-store porcelain plates. I scream into my hands and realize that I don't need to muffle the screams anymore. I'm here where no one can hear me and where cancer can cower behind the trees that protect me. I stand on shaky legs and take the first plate. I hold it close to my chest and breathe in deeply. I remember the 9-year-old girl who drifted out of her body and hovered above the 44-year-old woman she had become the moment she was told she was riddled with blood cancer. I shake with an unidentified emotion and feel a heavy tear roll down my cheek, connecting with the lip of the plate. I breathe and throw the plate at the tree 20 feet from me. I watch it break into pieces and think, "I can do better than that." I pick up the second plate and throw harder. And the third and the fourth, and with every throw, I become stronger, and the tears become hotter. The guttural screams surprise me, but I take them on fully. I scream until my voice becomes raw and throw until my right arm becomes tired.

It takes me two minutes for this firestorm of porcelain to end. I collapse into a ball on the wet ground covered in moss, leaves, and pasty dirt. I'm used to this fetal position. I've found myself here in hospital showers, bedroom floors, and below the kitchen sink, where washing dishes takes my mind to dark places. I lay on my side, hold my knees tight, and press my cheek against the earth. Gravity holds me down, and Earth becomes a welcome bed. My body starts to release its tension, and I'm tired. My scratchy throat from screams, wet cheeks from tears, and shaky palms from nerves all begin to settle back into place. And I smile. I smile at my bravery, faith, and anger as I pursue a sense of release. And I'm proud of myself for taking part in this crazy spectacle that laughed in the face of blood cancer anger.

I will no longer hide behind anger and take the "I'm fine" route. My body will know my attempt before I do and will let me know through an unsettled heartbeat and increased adrenaline. That's not worth my cellular health. This is not to suggest that I'll be screaming at my children (more than usual) or aggressively throwing plates within the protection of trees. Instead, I will work through the anger rather than trying to suppress it on my own, because attempting to snuff out the fire of rage is a losing battle. You might think you have things under control until one little spark reignites the whole process, and often, the embers burn hotter and faster this time.

Getting angry is a natural and human response. However, it's how we handle the anger that's most important. Don't be afraid to cry in the shower and collapse into a puddle of tears. It's okay to seclude yourself within the safety of your room and scream into your pillow until you can't anymore. It's OK to stand at the edge of the ocean or lake, throw rocks into the water, and cry a million tears while releasing what you might not even know through them. We must do things so that our body has a natural outlet. Energetically, our body is screaming from the inside out for us to take the time to recognize the imbalance, but then take it a step further and allow anger to have this door of escape.

For years, I pushed away anger. I found myself becoming ashamed of such a deep-rooted feeling of hatred, jealousy, or the many other emotions associated with its power. Upon reflection, I did this because I was trying to be a good person. But trying to be good only weakened me physically because I chose to look past my body's simple need to accept and affirm where it was at.

Every summer, I take my kids to the same boardwalk. I know the boards well and the surroundings even better. I have memorized the tourist-seeking shops and the pizza joints taunting customers with pies, staring straight at them through the see-through glass of the counter. I've walked hand in hand with all my children down this boardwalk until, at some point, and often without realizing it, they no longer need my hand. I squeeze three times. "I love you." They squeeze four times back, "I love you, too." Our secret connection.

The occasional boardwalk game comes along this walk amidst the shops and overpriced pizza joints. One of these games is my favorite, though I have never played it. You get a ball. You aim for a plate, watch it fall, then win a prize. I won't ever play this game because the story in my head is better. It's not better because of the cathartic release that I imagine it to bring. It's better because I'm giving my body the best prize through the process. It no longer has to stuff down anger to the point where, energetically, it has to carry it for years to follow. That choice is not worth my health, and certainly not worth ignoring the most essential gift granted to all of us. Our knowing choice is to live in such a way that serves as the greatest prize. Ourselves.

Truth 16: Detach

Be selfish here. Selfish is necessary.

I spent lots of time at my grandfather's house as a child. And I loved it there. It felt safe. I knew the home well. The deep-set closet underneath the stairs was a nice hideout for my sister and me when Sunday dinners went too long. The attic bedrooms hold tiny treasures from when my mom and her siblings were young, including a secret door built into the wall, my grandfather said was for emergency purposes. Knowing the practicality of his work and the quality of his handiwork in building the house, I believed him.

His kitchen had a shelf in the cabinet where "survival food" was kept. This included a few varieties of candy. However, a staple in this collection was Hershey's bars. There were always Hershey bars, and he smiled when he handed me a whole bar. It was our little secret. I believed my mom never knew. But since she brought him grocery shopping weekly, I'm sure she put the dots together. I remember distinctly that the shelf below held boxes of shredded wheat. Who wants to eat shredded wheat? I guess older people. His backyard was simple, with just one tree and a swing on it—a swing he had made for his grandchildren. As tiny as his property was, I explored it, knew it well, and took pride in my connection.

It was a sweltering summer afternoon. I was wearing a green, terry cloth tank top. This detail is important in the memory. I was exploring the outside of his concrete garage. A narrow path outside the garage was bordered by a fence that separated it from the neighbor's property. I walked carefully along the path, likely just exploring to see if I could find berries or something. Then, I feel tiny, uncomfortable pricks on my skin, through my shirt, and the irritating bruises on my 7-year-old knees. And within seconds, I am covered with burrs. And the more I try to remove them, the more they multiply. My fingers become pink and heated as I try to remove each one at a time. The interesting thing in this soon-to-be analogy is that I couldn't remove clumps of them as quickly as I could remove one at a time. In hindsight, I'm sure there were not as many burrs covering me as I recall now. But in my seven-year-old brain, I felt trapped. I bent down and took a few off my shoelaces, still trapped in the bushes that kept me hostage.

And then it happened. My hair. They took to my hair like magnets to energy. Since I was a highly emotional child, I started to cry. I must have looked pathetic. There I was. Stuck next to the garage, fingers sore, knees scratched, terry cloth sucking in prey, hair filled with burrs, and crying. At some point, I mustered up the courage to power through and fight my way out, which was probably all of four feet.

I make my way into the house, feeling defeated. Grandpa did the best he could to help with the hair situation. And I created a memory that was powerful enough to remember because of how being trapped in the burrs made me feel on an emotional level.

As adults, we get used to living in the traps of life. Isn't it easier to avoid something we don't want to deal with instead of putting in the hard work to detach ourselves from it? Over time, these traps become normal, and we design our lives around what we don't know, which is as uncomfortable as our nervous system feels. These traps are silent. They are poison to our full potential. Because anything that holds us back physically, emotionally, or spiritually

125

has no right to infect us. If not recognized and dealt with in a mindful approach, you will give these traps power to the point where you can't discern the trap from what a release could feel like.

If I asked you to write down five things in life that you feel trapped in, I'm sure the answers would come quickly. These traps come in all sizes. They don't necessarily have to be big. Sometimes, the smaller ones are the most harmful. Feeling trapped in a relationship, a friendship, or a job is a significant concern. Others might include feeling trapped in unhealthy eating patterns, the inability to quit smoking, or feeling unmotivated to get to the gym. When pressed on a more personal level, I'm sure you have a list distinct to your well-being.

We are tempted by emotional traps every day. Taking on the emotional energy of others struggling is not our responsibility. It is theirs to work through. As I continue to make my way through the healing process of being 18 months out from a bone marrow transplant, this has likely been the hardest truth for me to learn. The truth is to detach from the emotional needs and discontent of others. You are not responsible for their journey or the moments of enlightenment or discontent they experience. They are. The ironic part is that if I *do* make the unhealthy choice of stepping in every time they fall, I am disrupting the learning process for them and, at the same time, taking energy away from myself. There is no victory for either party and, more importantly, no growth.

Although many things in life can infect us with irrational thoughts and negative thinking, one of the most powerful influences is the company we keep. And whether it's a work colleague, a friendship, or a marriage partner, relationships are complicated. Most of us dance around the uncomfortable in these relationships because who wants to ruffle feathers? Well, I'm here to tell you, friends...get ruffling.

Take a complete inventory of the relationships in your life and decide which ones occupy too much emotional space. Which ones feel balanced? Which ones are just plain exhausting? Then, make a conscious decision to detach a bit from the ones that don't align with your needs. Be selfish here.

Selfish is necessary. If a friend needs you more than you need that friend, take a step back. I'm not suggesting you toss the relationship aside, but rather make yourself a priority. And since we are highly energetic beings, your friend will likely sense the change in you. And that's when you ruffle with love. You share gently the imbalance you feel. And inside your beautiful body, your soul celebrates you. Your cells multiply robustly with life because you are honoring YOU! You are not appeasing with quiet resentment toward the other person. You are making yourself the most important.

The tricky part is that most people won't understand your behavior. They are too self-absorbed, have a limited capacity for introspection, and are unwilling to take a baby step toward improving who they are in the presence of others. These individuals can still be part of your circle, but they are not your true friends. And when you begin creating space in that beautiful circle, you will be amazed at the kaleidoscope of souls that twinkle on in.

Detach from that person you know you should not be associated with. Detach from working extra hours to avoid what you should be looking at. Detach from family members who will never accept you and who you are meant to be. Detach from jobs that are mundane, unfulfilling, and exhausting. Detach from the things that don't feel right. It's that simple. They don't feel right. Listen to that. It's not quiet. It's loud. Those are the things you detach from.

And you don't do this quickly. You don't take a handful of burrs off your green terry cloth robe of life. You do this carefully. One burr at a time. The more you scramble, the more frantic you become to make significant changes, and the less space you give the universe to work alongside you. You will come out a bit scratched up and tired. That's okay because the scrapes of burrs are far less painful than the scars of unhealthy attachments.

Truth 17: Strong Is a Choice

And though the feeling of choosing strong amidst trial might feel foreign and scary, I promise you it will get easier.

Some choices are hard. Some are easy. Like most life lessons, both simple and complex, we learn this one as we become independent around age two. As quoted by Verruca Salt in Charlie and the Chocolate Factory, "I want it, and I want it now." At that age, we want what we want, and we want it now. However, over the years of mentally exploring the outcomes of our choices in both immediate and long-term contexts, we begin to realize that we have more ownership than we initially thought.

The easy and everyday choices: cookies and cream ice cream or mint chocolate chip? Should we go to the gym today? Wake up early on Sunday or choose to sleep in? Should I take the trip, or should I save the money?"

And as we well know, the more challenging choices hold a much heavier weight of possible repercussions or beauty. "Should I leave my job of 8 years because I'm unhappy and having a hard time with my colleagues? Should I attend an AA meeting or continue finding clever places in the house to hide my bottles? Should I leave the marriage that has me bound, even if it means pushing the real me into a corner of loneliness and a weighted blanket on my light?"

We face these complex and easy choices daily, and the older we get, the more we understand how hard this life is. We move through seasons of joy, sorrow, and loneliness, as well as carefree college days when time seems limitless and independence is discovered.

I watch my beautiful, powerful 17-year-old girl discover love for the first time. It's sweet, it's innocent, and she smiles a lot. Just like she did on her 5th birthday when she opened Sophia the First's Vanity. It fills my heart with joy to see her live in all her joy-filled self. Her prom is approaching this week, and her energy is light as she anticipates nail and hair appointments. Pictures with friends and a night every little girl looks forward to as much as her wedding day. It's the same energy that little girls' dress-up tea parties hold. The prom energy is just an extension of that meant to feed the princess in all of us.

I paused recently in my kitchen and took a moment to look at her. Somberly but joyfully remembering all of our sweet times spent together when she was little. The baking days, the park days, the American Girl Doll days, the princess outfit days that took trips to Target with us. And I said to myself that these days are not over. They are just different. She looked at me with the typical annoyed teenage angst and said, "What, mom?!" My eyes were a bit teary, but she didn't notice. "Honey, this is a great time of your life." She smiled, no words, and I was glad she was sinking into my words.

I know that hard choices are coming for her down the road. It's unavoidable in this life. However, one of the greatest lessons I want my children to learn is that when faced with difficult times, they are also given the power to choose how they will respond.

Being strong through a trial isn't something our mind just expectantly does. It's there in all of us. This silent power is just brewing beneath the surface. And as we feel the bubbles of fire rise, the more we tend to turn away. We don't trust our strength. We don't trust our strength because we don't practice it enough. And even more, our strength can scare us because once we step into the power of who we are, we aren't used to it. It is as though, through time and consistency, we can build the physical body through devotion to exercise. The mind is no different. Physical results show that pants fit better, sleep improves, and confidence increases.

Mental strength is felt. And the beautiful part is that once you recognize the power to choose strength over surrender, it becomes addictive. Your entire body sees your efforts and applauds you for standing in your truth and diving into what seems like jumping off a diving board thirty feet high.

I've lived most of my life living in this truth. And I'll continue strengthening my mental muscles with the challenges that come my way. And I encourage you to do the same. And though the feeling of choosing strong amidst trial might feel foreign and scary, I promise you it will get easier. You will start to see yourself as separate from those around you, as you no longer need to rely on the advice of others as much as you used to. You will build the growing awareness that you will not just grow on your journey if you trust your intuitive and mental strength. You will blossom.

One of my favorite children's books, which I read to my Kindergarten class, is a simple one with a powerful message. It's often the simple ones that have the best lessons. "Leo the Late Bloomer," written by Robert Kraus. A little tiger who can't keep up with his forest friends in their budding capabilities to read, write, jump, and dance. He is sad, watching from afar as their progress seems to come with ease. He practices, waits, and waits steadily for his day to come. And it does. Then, the book feels lighter, and the reader also feels the relief in Leo. We are the Leos, and we will all blossom in our own time when it comes to practicing our strength to change, move on, or face life's messy challenges while wearing armor we might hide behind but are willing to put on. And that's what matters. The very first step is to step into the armor.

I lay lonely in my bed, surrounded by the constant cricket sounds of machines beeping alongside me.

I squeeze my eyes shut and think of white sands and sunny skies somewhere across the world while a giant needle pushes and turns through my hip bone during multiple biopsies.

I struggle to swallow food without throwing it up or feeling like smashing my phone to pieces after FaceTime calls with my babies.

Or trusting for 90 days that a donor would come along.

All of these moments required strength.

And I didn't allow the alternative. Because the opposite of strong is weak. I was damned even to utter that word to my already disintegrating body. I chose to be strong in the thousands of moments this journey felt hard. I didn't question, "Why me?"...ever. It didn't enter my mind. I chose to believe that I had a greater purpose here. I didn't know what it was, and I still don't. However, if we live through strength, I promise that your efforts will not be in vain. You will be an encouragement to others without even realizing it. You will build a store of treasure in your soul where you can reflect and say, "Self...you did it then, you can do it now."

You can tell a lot about a patient on the bone marrow transplant floor when you glimpse their room. And I was given many opportunities to take a glance at rooms without being nosy. There wasn't much to look at during my monotonous walks with Hector as my buddy along hospital corridors. Hector, my vital machine, was a trustworthy, annoying friend that I had to keep around to stay alive. Some days, he administered cancer-killing drugs. On other days, magnesium drips or saline. He had good nights and bad nights. The bad nights included glitches in tubing, causing constant beeping and interrupted sleep. While Hector and I took our daily walks, I noticed that the patients who were bedridden or not doing their required daily walks were no longer there.

Some rooms have snacks, the shades are opened, and the patient eats in a chair with the side table pulled up close. These rooms were hopeful. Pictures of loved ones were placed along the window ledge, and the curtain and door were open. It was an invitation to visitors, even though we all knew we weren't allowed in each other's rooms because of infection. We followed that rule well, not because we were afraid to get caught. But because we wanted to survive. These patients drew strength from the simplest ways they could think of. And trust me, when you are isolated from the world, have no fresh air, and are hooked up like a dog to a leash in a lonely backyard, you find as many hidden bones as possible.

And then there are the dark rooms. They stay dark. The blinds are closed, the curtain is pulled three-quarters shut, and the door is closed. You do not see these patients, but you see the blue light filter through the darkness as the TV represents pretend social interaction. And you feel sad for these patients. These regular people were doing all the regular things before their diagnosis. And all they can think is, "Why me? I can't do this. I can't be here anymore." And I know they believe the awful because we all were tempted to think the awful in surprising and unexpected ways during this journey through hell.

Friends, choose strength. Weak carries too much risk. Your body will celebrate you in magnificent ways. You are the creator of your painting: dark, tiny strokes or big, bright, bold, and risky strokes. Trust the process of your work. You don't need to know the outcome. That doesn't matter. Because if you go into trials with a plan, it's YOU deciding how it will turn out. The strongest strength is the loudest whisper you will ever hear.

Truth 18: Listen

The more you honor another human being, the more you honor yourself.

Unfortunately, we live in a world that doesn't support our need to practice listening as much as we once did. Siri does what we tell her, and Alexa lights up when she hears her name. When we have a question, we ask a device or search for it, and within seconds, we have our answer. It's hard to imagine a life without devices that handle a significant amount of mental work. Before the rapid rise of technology, people interacted with one another.

This interaction was facilitated through conversation over a fence, an intentional phone call that didn't go to voicemail, or a handwritten letter in the mail. And these conversations were authentic. They were genuine because they challenged us (and still do) to study body language and facial expression, and we find ourselves navigating the energy of where the conversation goes. Technology serves as a cloak to the conversation. We communicate, but we can hide so much about how we feel when absent from the physical and vocal vibrations of another human on the other end. And through this slow decay of communication, we have lost the sweet art of listening. Just listening.

In my yoga teacher training program, I incorporate an exercise called "active listening." It involves a pair of students facing one another eye to eye. One person talks for five minutes about anything they want. The other partner listens, tries to maintain eye contact (which is challenging in and of itself), and is aware of facial expressions that could steer the conversation away from the topic at hand. I have not met one person who feels comfortable in either role. It's an incredibly uncomfortable exercise. I include this portion of my teacher training for students to learn how to get into their listening self, rather than planning their next thought based on someone else's idea. Teaching yoga is centered around listening. You listen to your breath, the room's energy, the vibrations of held poses, and actively listen to students who speak with you after class. This is the most beautiful part of teaching yoga, as it resonates with the energy felt during class. Watching your students grow into their bodies instead of growing out of them.

When we actively listen in a conversation, we are just listening. We aren't planning what we will say to steer the conversation toward ourselves. We prioritize the other person's words and ideas while supporting them in continuing their thought process. Too often, we interrupt too soon, and then, unaware, we selfishly take away their power to follow their thoughts to fruition.

I'm not suggesting we stare blankly at the other person without our own ideas brewing. What I'm suggesting is that we start the process of being introspective when in conversation. Understand that the other person chose you to talk to. Whether they invited you in or vice versa, it's a human-to-human connection, the most important connection. Respect that and respect the ideas of others. You will have your turn to talk; be patient. And when you respond, it doesn't always have to steer in your favor.

The truth here is that the more you honor another human being, the more you honor yourself. It is an act of humbling ourselves and loving someone else through the art of listening. When we love this way, we soften our hearts, remove the walls of superiority, and connect more deeply to who we are. So, in the end, it's a win-win. You love through listening, and in turn, you soften. And your cells learn through listening that they can take their guard down and stop working so hard to fight their way to the front and take over. They are happy to rest in your love for yourself and others.

Listening through conversation and vibrational exchange is the most immediate form we can begin practicing, as it's tangible and allows us multiple daily opportunities to practice. However, a form of listening runs deep in all of us. And if we allow ourselves to be a bit more reflective and vulnerable, we will find that all the answers we need are immediately and always within us. And when awakened and given power, they can guide you one trusting thought at a time. This might not seem very easy and may be a bit esoteric. But if you step away from your regular routines and schedules and get quiet with your visions and deepest desires, you will begin to discover, through patience, that your body has much to tell you.

Listening from the inside out works with where you are at in your current state. Listening from the outside intends to inform you from another's perspective what you should be doing and how you should be doing it, and it will likely interrupt your body's brilliant intuitive self. Start small. Don't expect big answers. Just start listening to what your inner professor has to say. The tiny morsels of wisdom you begin to discover when fed with quiet respect begin to grow, and as they grow, they build your confidence in trusting yourself.

I practice this truth every day. All day. When my five-year-old, stuffy-nosed kindergarten students hand me another picture of a rainbow to add to my collection of 100s, I look them in the eye and listen to them. How they made it, where they made it, and why they made it. This affirms them; it takes accolades away from me, and they leave feeling loved. I sense their subtle frustration as they try to grasp concepts that come easily to the students next to them, but not to them. I listen when I'm in a conversation with an individual whom I immediately don't trust. I've become good at this one. That energy runs deep, and pangs of flashing lights steer me away gently. I listen to what I should be doing even if I don't want to. The more I listen and become quiet, the more I discover and the more opportunities I give myself to move forward with prosperity and health.

On July 12, 2022, I stood at my kitchen sink washing dishes with a terrible pain on my left side. I had a slight fever and was feeling tired. I had already been to urgent care the day before, and the doctor assured me that I was anemic and had to increase proteins, such as red meat. I stopped washing dishes and looked out the window. I was scared. My body was telling me something. And I couldn't stop listening. My breath was shallow, and I found myself deep in the trenches, needing answers to something my body couldn't contain anymore.

I looked at my beautiful middle girl, who stood next to me, pouring a bowl of cereal while watching TikTok. The one that I say every year on her birthday, "One of the best parts about a sandwich is the middle." And I say through wet eyes, "Stella, something is wrong with me." Without a pause, she looks up and says, "Mom, go to the hospital. You need to." I went. And I didn't stand at my kitchen sink until 49 days later. Stella listened. I listened. And my body saved my life even while it was dying.

October 2022: A Dancing Queen

October resembles most of September's routines. I'm starting to feel like a mom again. Grocery lists come more naturally, and breaking up sibling fights seems less exhausting. I continue to wait in limbo, along with the innate knowing that a donor is still out there. I wonder sometimes if this is my body's way of masking the reality that there might not be someone who can save my life. Either way, there is nothing I can do about it. I'm a sitting duck just waiting for an answer.

In the meantime, I mindlessly escape my worries with frequent outings with friends. It's the time of year on the Jersey shore when October's weather can sometimes replicate the weather of June. Bars still have outdoor seating, and locals know where to avoid on Friday nights. I take on the mindset of "What the hell? I might die anyway." It's not a mindset I chose. In retrospect, I felt like it found me. And I didn't push it away. I just welcomed it because I didn't give a fuck. At this point, I was still waiting for a phone call. And it wasn't a call about getting a job or a routine breast exam result. It was a call that would determine whether or not I might zip up my daughter's wedding dress or see my grandchildren someday.

I love to dance. I always have. It's similar to a moving meditation, but only works if the dancer dances without abandon. The music, the smells, the noise, and the atmosphere create a bubble that's all your own. It's a Friday night at a popular bar in town. I'm wearing a green sweater. I chose it because I'm told that green brings out the color in my eyes. I walk into this night without rules. I'm going to dance, I'm going to drink, I'm going to make new friends, and pretend that blood cancer was never a part of me. My plan works. I clear the floor. I'm good, and others watch with envy as I move fluidly to the music. A young man walks into my circle and joins my eight-count rhythm perfectly. He's a stranger, I'm a stranger, but music brings it all together. It becomes a dance beyond a dance. People fade into the noise, and it's just him and me, feeling an energy that others admire. I tried to embody the sensations as much as possible because I wanted to write about this moment. It was significant as I lived to my fullest without a care. How could any care be bigger than the care of waiting for a bone marrow donor?

My night continues with my new friend. A decision was made at a time when escaping was at its peak. I didn't care, and I didn't want to care. I was in a place where I didn't want to feel anything. I knew exactly what I was doing, so I justified my behavior with the awareness of my poor decision. In retrospect, I know what it looked like. A 40-something feeling attractive and sexy while awaiting a fate that would determine the rest of her life. This man was just a convenient drug that brought a momentary high. I didn't regret my decision the next day. Instead, I pictured other moms in town talking about me. And I liked the vision I came up with. People often criticize others for making bad decisions because they have had similar desires themselves. But they aren't close enough to death to dabble in the game of "Who gives a fuck."

It's a Tuesday, and Tuesdays often mean a routine visit to Hope Tower. I've always felt bad for Tuesday. It's the day of the week that doesn't have a purpose like the other days. Monday is the beginning, Wednesday is the middle, and Thursday is the anticipation for everyone's favorite day. Friday is the popular kid in the class, and Saturday is the cool cousin. Sunday is Sunday. It's a low-key, regroup kinda of day. The only thing Tuesday has going for it is the two-for-one specials at pizza joints. Business owners know that most people aren't ordering out mid-week, especially on the day that is the most mundane of them all. But Tuesdays are important to me.

Every Tuesday, I visit Hope Tower, meaning I'm one week closer to complete healing. It's the same feeling I get when I have to fill my weekly medicine box. It's a process I loathe, but I love it all at the same time. This task takes concentration and time. My kids know not to interrupt me when I'm counting out pills and making notes on previous discharge sheets concerning dosages. I line up the 14 bottles of various colored pills, all shapes and sizes. I am not confident enough to do this without my cheat sheet. One misstep, and I leave a note out of the symphony that's taking place within the cellular walls of my body.

This Tuesday morning is a beautiful Fall morning. Harvest-colored flowers and cornstalks are newly placed at the hospital doors. I've come to appreciate the people who change the hospital's decor according to the seasons. When you are a patient whose second home is this building, you start to notice the changes and appreciate the tiny details that staff take to keep spirits up, even if it means a cute scarecrow bought from The Christmas Tree Shop.

I take the short elevator ride up to the 2nd floor. The Leukemia and Bone Marrow Transplant floor. I step into a waiting room of my fellow fighters and take in the same smells, noises, and feelings. Most of us are quiet, but we all come with someone by our side, except for me. I've come to 90% of my appointments alone. Doctors

141

and nurses see my loneliness and watch me scribble notes on my yellow legal paper pad as quickly as possible. I don't have someone here to listen to the doctor's weekly updates or review the tedious meds list. They have become my family, my sisters, and my mothers. They know the details of my life outside these walls. They know that my girls play soccer and that my twins are two completely different personalities.

Violet, a born intuitive, overflows with love. Her sea-blue eyes beam, and she is learning that all the love she has to give doesn't always save the day the way you want it to. Charlie, a natural inventor, creator, and external thinker, balances out Violet's dreamer type. They know that my oldest is surviving his first year of college. They know what shows I like to watch and which boardwalks I enjoy walking on. I used to think that hospital staff made patient connections out of obligation. Instead, I've realized over these past several weeks that they genuinely care. I know that they "see" me as a life they want to continue saving. I am one of the reasons they chose this profession, and I firmly believe that those entrusted with my care value life and health above all other professions.

I wait for my nurse to visit and review the extensive list of my medications. I appreciate this part of the appointment. We collaborate to ensure I take the proper medications and dosages on the correct days. It's become a routine I've excelled in, but I am careful never to handle this portion of the appointment lightly. Once the medication list is complete, my nurse puts down her pad and smiles at me. It's a smile I haven't seen from her yet. It's a different smile. And since we all wear masks, I can only see her eyes smiling, but it's a good smile. After a slight pause, she says, "Congratulations, I'm so happy for you." Her eyes smile a little brighter with each word. I'm a little confused. *Were my blood counts better than normal? What does she know that I don't know?* She notices my non-reaction and quickly fills the silence. "You have a donor, and it looks like a great match." Her voice becomes faint as she trails off, explaining how the doctor will discuss this in more detail. The external noises from the hallway continue to grow quieter. I can see her talking, but I can't process what she's saying. My breath feels light, and my heart races slightly, but races with happy beats instead. Blood rushes from my face, and I want to cry a little. But I want to save the tears for my car parked in the Walgreens parking lot. I don't want to share these happy tears with anyone but myself. The nurse leaves the room and smiles again as she closes the door.

My Doctor and the nurse manager entered the room a few minutes later. They share the same excitement but are much more subdued. They share this moment with me but know from their experience that my fate falls within the steps taken to prepare for the transplant and the recovery to follow. I'm eager to learn more about the details of my donor. Is my donor male or female? Where are they from? How old are they? What is their story? I can tell my doctors anticipate these questions as I'm a newbie BMT patient. They told me my donor was a 26-year-old male who weighed 224 pounds. It is not confirmed where he is from, but the letterhead on the hospital paperwork suggests that he is from Germany.

I take a moment to visualize what my donor looks like. He is tall, strong, and likes his beer. He's a good man, and his mother raised him right. He has many friends and works as a barista at a local coffee shop until he finds a job related to his recent master's degree. Environmental Engineering. I imagine that he receives a phone call while making a cranberry-spiced latte. He allows the call to go to voicemail and checks the message while on break. He listens to the voicemail two more times. He's not sure what to make of this news. A 44-year-old female in the United States requires a bone marrow transplant, and he's her match. He recalls getting swabbed at a college fair when he was 18. He didn't know what being on a bone marrow registry meant, but all his buddies were doing it, so he felt he should be, too. Besides, the table provided decent chocolates; he felt bad about taking the chocolate without being swabbed.

I bring back my swirling imagination to the present moment. I collect myself and try to act as professionally as possible. My doctor shares the many steps I need to take before the transplant. I scribbled notes and carefully organized all scripts, referrals, medication, and discharge papers in the well-worn blue and white folder I was first handed upon admission to Jersey Shore Hospital in July. The folder is shredded at the seams and edges. It is decorated with scribbles of doctors' names and random phone numbers on the front and back covers. Doodle marks and a few emails are part of the visual chaos. I still carry this same folder to all of my present-day doctor appointments. It's just held together with duct tape. It's kind of how I feel as I await my transplant.

The weeks following the news of my donor are spent preparing for my transplant. My weeks are filled with every precautionary test imaginable: respiratory tests, scans, thorough dental work, and consultations with various specialists. My body must be ready for battle as it anticipates the war it's about to enter. I take each appointment in stride. I take pride in my organization in all of this and admire myself for doing it on my own. It's me, my folder, and my doctors. We are the only ones aware of how lengthy and exhausting this process is.

When I reflect on the weeks preceding my transplant, I feel as though I'm watching a professional woman who is determined not to make one mistake. I don't want to miss one appointment, pill, or moment to thank the visiting nurse who changed my port weekly in my home. I never allowed myself to doubt the impending procedure that would save my life.

There was never a moment I allowed myself to listen to the faraway lie that I might not be here next year. I was self-aware enough to understand that I wouldn't be human if I didn't often have these dark and haunting thoughts at the most inconvenient times. They crept up in the middle of the night or when I received transfusions, amidst 50 other sick patients who surrounded me. My thoughts were challenged, and I was irritated. I was damned to allow anything to mess with my strength.

I saw cancer as something that was outside of me and not a part of me. I laughed at it and rolled my eyes, which worked because it made me the boss. The cancer had to report to me, and cancer knew that this boss wouldn't take shit. It tried to threaten, scare, shock, and blindside me, but I stood firm and continued to. I gripped my hospital bed rails during bone marrow biopsies, gritted my teeth, and watched my knuckles turn white. And the harder I squeezed, the smaller the cancer became.

I walked out of Hope Tower that Tuesday in a daze. I didn't use the crosswalks to cross the parking lot. I barely looked up. Cars stopped, and drivers were annoyed. I didn't care. I felt invincible now that I had a donor. My pace picked up as I neared the Walgreens parking lot. My black Tahoe was my safety. I climbed in, closed the door, and screamed. It was a mix of anger, joy, and relief all at once. I plunged my head forward, and it rested on top of the steering wheel. I watched the tears roll down the center of the wheel. I shook, I hugged myself tight, and I repeated two words over and over again. "Thank you, thank you, thank you." I don't know how long I stayed in my cave or who I was thanking. Was it God? My donor? I believe both. I just knew that now I had a chance to zip up my daughters' wedding dresses someday.

Truth 19: Be Conscious, Not Careless

Yes, you are worthy child.

I don't trust people. I know that sounds harsh, but I don't. I'm still working on unpacking where this stems from in my weekly therapy appointments, and I'm sure that someday I'll start to understand why. But, for now, I still keep my guard up. I am cautious in conversation. I am selective about what I say and with whom I discuss things. I've learned throughout my adult life that people often prioritize their interests, even if that means hurting others in the process. We are all still very much like children in this way. Most of us do things unknowingly to serve our interests. I want to believe this is a form of a deep-seated survival mechanism that we can't help. Or instead, an unconscious selfish reaction to get what we want and get it now. And that's a very human and natural response.

And there are hidden parts of us that we dare not expose to one another. Those are the aspects of people that make me nervous and cause me to retreat into my shell of self-preservation. When I don't trust people, the word "cautious" needs to be slightly tempered. I need to work on this, but I share my flaw to encourage you to be cautious about who you associate with and understand that the word "trust" is defined differently for some.

When we walk across streets, we look both ways. We do this intuitively because an adult lovingly instilled this in us when we were young. The adult was teaching us how to protect ourselves. When we turn left in a car, we look both ways several times because we took a driver's ed. course that taught us the rules of driving to protect ourselves. We wash our hands, wear seat belts, and do millions of other things daily for some protection. We learn to be cautious in the basics of life to protect who we are. We mostly learn cautious practices to protect our physical bodies. However, I want to delve into how to be mindful when protecting our mental and spiritual well-being.

A verse in the bible says, "Avoid the appearance of evil." (1 Thessalonians 5:22) I've never liked this verse, as it was often used as a form of parenting for me while growing up, mainly during my teenage years. It made me feel that others' perspectives of me were more important than the choices I would have to take ownership of. The verse instructs us not to associate with people or practices that could appear to present sinful behavior on the outside. Maybe God was trying to protect us with these words, but I didn't resonate with them because they diminished my judgment to make conscious and good choices. I wondered in my teenage brain, "How am I going to help the *bad* people if I can't be seen with them?" It was all very confusing for me, but as I read scripture now through the lens of life experience and unjaded awareness, I can sift through the nuances that bound me. Furthermore, I find strength in knowing that these words don't have the power to suffocate who Christ designed me to be.

I value scripture and believe it is "God-breathed," as the Christians say. I am grateful for the hundreds of verses I have stored in my memory bank, thanks to Bible summer camps, youth groups, and Sunday school projects. These verses are always quick and ready for me; I consider them golden words. I cling to the verses filled with love, peace, encouragement, and hope. I am aware of the verses that are soaked with condemnation, judgment, and shame. The twisted part about being raised in my faith was the way that I seemed to put a greater emphasis on the fear-inflicting scriptures versus the ones that soothe and heal. So, I learned to live in fear of the condemnation of Christ's wrath if I wasn't a good Christian girl. I

n the early days of my diagnosis, I believed I was being punished for choices that didn't line up with the Christian girl script. I realized I was conditioned to fall back on this untrue script because that made the most sense. The crazy part is that I found some comfort in it all. Is that the same thing as one who's abused returning to their abuser? In the world of Psychology, this is referred to as trauma bonding. My bonding was my faith.

I am now aware of how to be in my body. How do we discern what judgment is and what shame is? I can put up invisible shields of protection to protect myself emotionally. I have learned that God is love. And that's it. He's simply love. He is not a God of fear. He doesn't tower over us with a trident reflecting that of King Triton in The Little Mermaid. And if we recall that beautiful story, we remember how much the King loved his baby girl at the end. And that's how I believe my God sees me.

Living carelessly means believing what we are told without being curious enough to understand why it affects us the way it does. Living carelessly means trusting too many people and not yourself. You are more powerful than you know. And I don't think I can write this message any better with any other words. Trust me, I've tried to figure out how to convey better that you ARE the power. But you won't feel or step into your power unless you let the reins go a bit. Those reins hold back your spirit. When you are conscious of your choices and interactions daily, you give the Universe or God the open door to work through and with you. The more we try to control, the more careless we are. Control means taking the reins and steering. Conscious awareness means being vulnerable and trusting the process of where we are headed. In some ways, it's a backward way of thinking. We consider control to be the pilot's responsibility. On course, steady, and consistent.

In this case, control takes away your intuitive "knowings" of what your body is telling you. And those intuitive "knowings" are the perfect set of directions for your life. We are scared of the truths because we don't believe we can live up to them or, more so, attempt them. This is where the rubber meets the road. Do you trust yourself to find the answers within yourself? They are always there, within a millisecond of being asked. But the problem is the chatter. The outside noise gets in the way of making the next move that could benefit you. The bottom line here is that you need to trust yourself. Not your background, not what you think you want, not what others "suggest" you should do. You were designed to be someone. And that someone is someone powerful and deserving. Yes, you are deserving!

I've lived my whole life with difficulty. Seven years battling a relentless eating disorder, pressure to perform in my athletic endeavors throughout high school and college, navigating mental health in a variety of relationships, birthing a dead baby, overworking, and living in a loveless marriage. I share my "hard" to invite you to believe that you deserve the good as much as I do. But that good doesn't find you and can't see you until you surrender to it and allow it to float through the doors of your heart. And when you feel that little light inside of you that says, *Yes, you are a worthy child*, it's there that you start to fan the flame in the smallest ways that you can. It might be baby pep talks, looking in the mirror and telling yourself how awesome you are, or perhaps just taking a moment to breathe and be grateful for the good things around you.

When you live consciously and are fully aware of what you are meant to be and have, you make way for the good to float in. And be ready because once you make this a daily habitual way of thinking, you will have difficulty keeping up with all the good. I promise you! Life wants to serve you the most delicious meal you have ever tasted. Don't carelessly glance at the menu and order what you always do, because it's familiar and safe. Let the waiter suggest one of the chef's specials. And when you introduce and enlighten your taste buds with something they didn't know was available, you will never have to look at another menu again. You will trust the environment around you.

Truth 20: Accept It

We have to choose to accept the hard.

I am reminded daily of life post-cancer. These reminders are subtle at times. For example, I fill my pill box on Sunday nights, where I'm careful not to make a mistake—washing my hair with expensive biotin shampoo and weekly rosemary oil hair masks, willing it to grow. And then there are the heavy reminders. I have debilitating neuropathy pain in my hands and feet on hot days because of Chemotherapy treatments. Hiding behind SPF 50 hats in the summer and lathering in expensive sunscreen makes me feel like a pale toddler on the beach. This protects my skin from flaring up with graft vs. host disease—a severe condition for bone marrow patients for the rest of my life. And the monthly reminder of blood draws is examined by the doctor for any slight detectable signs of cancer creeping back in.

I've joked through this process that I'm a china doll and must be handled carefully. One little crack in my smooth, porcelain cellular self could cause everything to come crashing down into a thousand pieces.

I've struggled with accepting my body post-cancer. I have found myself willing my strong and faithful body to be like it was pre-cancer. The result just led me to get angry with cancer and continue to tell it that I was in charge. But the problem with this way of thinking when recovering from what I've been through is that you are extending so much extra undo energy and unknowingly giving cancer a little bit of power.

This realization came to me when I was driving home from a recent and spontaneous doctor's appointment where I unexpectedly had to go in for bloodwork as my blood draws two days prior looked suspicious. And that's the most challenging part about blood cancer. You never really feel as though you are in the clear. I went through all my go-to emotions of anger, frustration, and exhaustion with these appointments two years out from diagnosis! And while lost in conflicting emotions at a stoplight, I pull down the mirror above me. I looked into my own eyes, and I saw a different person. And in some weird, energy-driven way, I accept for the first time that my body will never be the same as it was before diagnosis. And the most unexpected feeling followed soon after. Release. A sigh of relief, a surrender, a knowing that I don't have to try to be who my former self was. 2

If I'm completely transparent, I don't want to return to that version of Sarah. She was drinking to survive, overworking to survive, numbing through unhealthy emotional connections to survive, and trying to fight loneliness to survive. All the while, my survival techniques were the very things that were slowly killing me. And I smile in the mirror and shake my head slightly, dropping it in self-surrender. I am in awe of this healing process. It's ever-changing and surprising. And I'm learning through it all that all I have to do is accept what's here. What's here now. At the moment. And that has been one of the biggest lessons of all. A truth I will continue to practice to feel that cathartic relief over and over again.

We have to choose to accept the hard. The changes and unexpected potholes along the way. Some things we can change. Others we can't. And the more we try to push away the hard or, worse yet, ignore it, the louder it becomes.

If you define your life with negativity, it's winning already. Don't let it win. You are in charge of how you speak in the face of challenge. Your cells crave your acceptance and honesty in respecting yourself enough to accept what is there and what you cannot change. Those cells are working hard enough to keep you healthy. They don't want to have to deal with your negative thinking.

From the very moment I heard the word *Leukemia*, *diagnosis*, and *Sarah* in the same sentence, I decided that cancer would not define me. I was stuck in a deep, dry well surrounded by what didn't look like there was much of a way out. I didn't scramble; I didn't Google; I tried not to dwell on blood tests and their results. But instead, I chose to accept where I was. And in that acceptance, I felt as though I created space for healing. Don't get me wrong, I had massive emotional tantrums along the way, but I always chose to look at cancer in its ugly face and accept its presence in my body.

People cocked their heads and never understood why I didn't wear a wig when I lost my hair. I chose not to wear one because cancer wanted me to feel ugly with no hair. If I chose a wig, I felt like I was giving in to cancer's lies and, therefore, it resulted in cancer winning. I accepted I had no hair and chose to feel beautiful without it, realizing how pretty, flashy, dangly earrings made me feel.

Acceptance is not easy. And it's not easy, over and over again. It becomes something we practice, and something many of us fail at. We fail because the hard thing we are trying to accept is hard to embody. Please notice the feelings that arise when you work through the acceptance process. What is there? Anger, fear, guilt, shame, embarrassment? Those are the things that require effort to help us strive toward the ultimate goal of complete acceptance. I must accept that my life will never be the same as it was before July 15, 2022. I must accept that my future birthdays will hold more significance for me than they have in the first 44 years of my life. I must accept that low-lying fear will permanently reside in dusty corners of my brain, but it's up to me to dust those corners occasionally.

This all brings me to a different kind of acceptance. The understanding that we deserve good things. I deserve good things. I still look back on my journey and have difficulty accepting that I came through this difficult time. And I struggle with questioning why others did not.

A friend I had come to know throughout my treatment was a light in my life. She would share texts of encouragement and quotes with me as she was about six months ahead of me in her healing process. We compared blood results and chemotherapy side effects and joked that we were sexy vampires who had become blood experts. She was beautiful in ways that I cannot put into words. Her funeral was one of the hardest I have ever attended.

Sometimes, life makes no sense, and we can either wallow in these nagging questions or focus on the good we are experiencing now. We must choose that we are worthy of good things coming our way —a truth I still try to embrace daily. Our body wants to celebrate us. It wants us to breathe these beautiful moments of daily and unexpected joy. Instead of waiting for the next shoe of life to drop, look at your closet full of sparkly, red-bottomed heels!

When we accept *ALL* of who we are, the blessings and heartaches we give our bodies are some of the best gifts. We can celebrate the joys and heal by accepting "the hard." Choose joy. Choose surrender. Choose to melt into the truth that you are worthy. You are worthy because you are a child of God. God is love. Your body craves to be enveloped in as much love as possible.

Truth 21: Just Love

When we love deeply during the most challenging times and with the most difficult people, we soften our hearts and love ourselves more deeply.

I am confident that love is a mystery to all of us. It's a mystery because it has many levels and winding, uncertain paths. It reminds me of the ancient Hindu Metaphor of Indra's Net. An intertwining net of jewels that are all interconnected with one another. Every action has a reaction that ripples through our beings, informing our thoughts, who we attract, and our choices. If the Indra's Net metaphor was sculpted by love, I wonder what it would look like. Start with one tiny jewel of love when we are born, and watch as the manifestation of what love can do unfolds when applied to every action and reaction. Love is a feeling, but one that is unique to each of us. Love is an action toward another. Love is forgiveness. Love is treating ourselves as necessary. Love is so many things. But to "just love," as simple as it sounds, might be their highest calling.

We've all been there—the neighbor who has passive-aggressive summer parties and plays their backyard music too loud at 1 am. The friend who seems inconsistent with support when you are going through something, you are there for them whenever they need you, or the relative who is critical, distant, and apathetic. There are countless scenarios of emotional frustration regarding the people in our lives whom we are challenged to love, especially those closest to us.

Reacting with frustrations and withholding love takes the briefest of moments to melt into. And when you melt here for too long, you eventually dissolve into not feeling much of anything for the other person. However, intuitively aware of our instant reactions in these cases matters most. It's practiced. It's practiced daily. Ask yourself, "How do I love this person when I feel slighted?" You do. You love. I'm not suggesting you become a doormat for other people's emotional shit. I'm offering a different perspective. On paper, this all sounds ridiculous. It sounds like we are bowing to the choices of others, weakening our spirits. This is not the case. You are doing the complete opposite. When we love deeply during the most challenging times and with the most difficult people, we soften our hearts and love ourselves more deeply.

As Johnny Cash is one of my favorite artists, Robin Williams is right up there with him. We all know his story, his heartache, and his fight with mental demons, which, in the end, were too big for him to conquer. And with Robin comes his infamous quote, which penetrates all of us on some level. It penetrates us because we resonate with pain. We resonate with the pain because we experience it in some form every day.

"Everyone you meet is fighting a battle you know nothing about. Be kind. Always."

- Robin Williams

And I wonder if Robin just wanted to be loved hard. If someone he trusted sat across from him, held him, listened to him, and loved him by just being there. We need to look past the fancy cars and expensive boats. We need not let the comments of the seemingly "perfect" mom get under our skin.

Here's a secret. They all want to be loved. The actions of others are not your shit. You can separate yourself from their energy and love them simultaneously. Don't get sucked into the gossip, the pity, and the judgment. Our cellular self doesn't want those kinds of stale nutrients. This does nothing for us. Our blood is flat, not vibrant. Our light is dim, not bright. To love is to forgive and to forgive quickly. To love is to extend grace and accept people as they are. Carry your ten-foot pole around. Know who you need to distance yourself from, but love them from afar.

I'm still trying to figure out what it means to love myself. My therapists have thrown this phrase around as if it's something I'm expected to understand. I'm working through it, feeling it at times and searching for it at other times. I've tried going out to dinner by myself. I've tried sleeping in on purpose. I've tried taking a day off of work just because. But none of this feels natural. It all feels forced. I know that loving myself will come naturally someday. I'm unsure what it will feel like, but the mini-changes I make along the way can't hurt. And if I'm honest... I struggle to love myself. I battle guilt and question if I was the reason my life imploded on me and my kids. I wonder if I'm lovable to other people. And I wonder if I will ever experience what it means to "be in love."

Thesis papers, books, and millions of studies have explored the concept of love in some capacity. But the irony is that when we apply this word to our lives, we don't know what to do with it. Maybe I'm not giving much advice or direction regarding this truth. And it's likely because I don't have the answers for myself. But I do know one thing. I know that when we love hard, we feel good. I know that when we see people as broken, we feel empathy. We feel empathy because we are human, and all humans feel this, whether or not they are vulnerable enough to verbalize it. Extending love to others is rooted in the soul of loving who we are— loving ourselves despite divorce, loving ourselves despite bad choices, loving ourselves despite mistakes, and loving ourselves when it feels like we are the most unlovable toy in the toy box of adulting.

When people challenge me on my faith, *how do you know there is a God? How do you know there is Heaven? Why do you go to church?* I've fielded hundreds of questions, all asking the same thing. Asking why, I believe. And for me, the answer is simple. I feel God's love every day. I feel Him leading me, providing for me, protecting me. I feel this love because I've been open to it. I don't need to memorize scripture, host bible studies, or volunteer for church nursery duties. That was pre-cancer, Sarah. God IS love. I was created in His image and, therefore, a walking embodiment of Him. And as it was written in the most popular text of creation.

1 Corinthians 13:13, Paul writes, "So now faith, hope, and love abide, these three; but the greatest of these is love."

This was read at my wedding as it's the go-to verse to include in 90% of wedding ceremonies. People read it because it sounds appropriate. It sounds light and pretty. But it's much more than that. Faith is believing that which is not seen. Hope is trusting the outcome to something unknown, and those two principles, in and of themselves, are a lot to unpack. But love surpasses both of them. That's powerful. Perhaps we struggle to love ourselves because love is a beautiful mystery that we are meant to unravel throughout our lifetime, until we encounter the creator of this thing called love. And the creator of this thing called love states, "The greatest of these is love." (1 Corinthians 12:13)

Truth 22: Energy is Honest

Our vibrational self can sense what's wrong before we clean up a mess we were too ignorant to avoid.

I was about seven years old when I first learned about energy. And I was caught off guard. I was too young to understand it, but I was wise beyond my years when I felt it.

Being raised in the "born-again" faith, believing in Santa Claus was not up for debate. There was no Santa. There was Jesus. He was "the reason for the season." The cherry-cheeked, red-suited, jolly ol' fella was to be enjoyed by my friends. I went along with holiday school songs and wrote letters to him, knowing they had found their way into my town's post office garbage, not the North Pole. The crazy part is that I was okay with all of this. I liked knowing this secret before all my other friends discovered the truth. Yet, despite all this, I wondered if a twinkling star on Christmas Eve was possibly his sleigh. Dabble with imagination; it will take you places, even for a fleeting moment.

I recall my first experience of reading energy with such clarity. And as I've mentioned before, we recall particular moments in life in detail when they've had a profound emotional impact on us.

Our family was at a neighbor's Christmas party. Parents mingled and expected us to play when we were just bored. I always thought that was funny about parents when I was a kid. They just expected that we were playing and not listening. I listened a lot. I entered the dining room, where the cookies and other holiday treats were on tier-level trays. Between the door from the kitchen and the dining room was a gentle-looking man sitting on a chair. He was older, and he had a drink in his hand. He looked at me and said, with a sweet smile and a slight lean forward, "Are you ready for Santa?" I just looked at him. He continued by asking what I hoped Santa would bring. I kept looking at him and didn't like how I felt. I stood a little straighter, looked him straight in his eyes, and said, "I don't believe in Santa." I walked away and immediately felt bad, thinking I might have hurt his feelings. Yet simultaneously, I was proud of myself for standing in my truth.I felt his energy was sincere, but I also sensed that it was pandering.

There I was. A small, bored child at an adult Christmas party. He saw my glazed-over eyes and cookie crumbs on my collar and wanted to cheer me up. He tried to connect with me. But he did the opposite. He pushed me away because I felt like he wasn't honoring me as someone I felt like I was. After spending the last 23 years working with children, I realized I was not the norm. But the flicker of pandering energy I felt in that 20-second exchange seeped deep into the well of who I was becoming and what this world was teaching me. Energy swept through my naive 65-pound body and taught me, for the first time, that there is a language bigger and more informing than any spoken language.

And since that first experience of feeling the emotional shift and self-awareness, I have learned one lesson. To trust energy because it's honest. I believe energy is felt by all of us in different ways. For some, it's an increased heart rate. For others, it is a pit in our stomachs. But for all of us, it comes down to a "knowing" when we are still enough and okay with who we are. This "knowing" is hard to describe because words aren't always great at capturing the nuances that weave through us in the most unexpected ways.

Over time, I've learned to listen to energy as deeply as I listen to the people most important to me. And in many ways, listening with energy ears is far more potent than the physical processing of verbal exchange. I've also learned hard lessons when I haven't listened with my energy ears. I've been hurt, sucked into emotional abuse, and, most importantly, didn't recognize that energy was trying to protect me. And that's just it. Our vibrational self can feel what's not right before we clean up a mess we were too ignorant to avoid.

Like many truths in this book, discerning energy is challenging. It needs to be practiced. The practice is not just listening to it and feeling it. The practice is doing what energy is telling you to do. It's honest, it doesn't lie, it's pretty black and white. It's not complicated. Like so many other things in life, we humans are the ones who make it complicated. Don't overthink it or try to adjust the subtleties it's telling you. You have the answer. You know the answer. You are responsible for whether or not you will put on the available armor of protection.

This might sound like a foreign concept, but I get that. It sounds untouchable, likely because you are in a place where you do not want to tap into who you are and what you deserve. You might be putting up your armor of protection. And often, these protective devices are the unhealthy choices we make in life in order not to feel what we know we should be feeling, but knowingly avoid. We drink, we get involved in relationships we know are not good for us, we overeat, we take drugs, and the list goes on. The more we mindlessly suffocate our immense power to feel, the further we get away from who we are. And these actions are not fair to your cellular self. Trust me. I lived there for too long. I thought I had the answers figured out through the surface choices of protection I was coming up with. None of my ideas worked. They all backfired on me. And when they did, I tried other ways of self-preservation. And now, post-leukemia, I walk through life, taking down the curtains of what I thought could protect me. Now, the light comes straight in. Blinding at times, and I find myself seeking energy everywhere I go. And I feel my body healing from the inside out. And this is because I am finally honoring what I need to be healthy and, just as importantly, whole.

Start simple. Wake each morning and honor how you feel in the moment. If you feel sad, allow yourself to feel sad. Maybe you don't have an answer to why you are unhappy, depressed, anxious, etc., and that's okay. Just acknowledge it because by acknowledging it, you are owning it. You are taking the first step toward listening with energy ears. You are affirming what your body teaches and helping you with it now. Then, the most magical and supernatural thing starts to happen.

Everywhere you go, you are sensing things you never sensed before. You figure out who you can trust and who you can't trust. That might be the most significant energy lesson to take away. People can make us feel lovely, or they can begin slowly deteriorating and dimming that blinding light coming in past the curtains.

Trust what you feel in every single moment. Honoring your energy is better than any organic and expensive supplement out there. Your body has all the answers. Please don't try to figure them out on your own. This never ends well. Ever.

Truth 23: Be a Truth Teller

It's like coming home when you can listen to your body and let go of the heavy stuff.

A verse in the bible says, "And you will know the truth, and the truth will set you free" (John 8:32). These words are easy to interpret on the surface level. Lies are hard to tuck away. Especially the ones we are ashamed of. They hold a dark tug on our hearts, and over time, we adapt to living with it, hoping that someday we will have the courage to cut it off and feel set free. We know this verse holds great wisdom. That's not up for debate. Yet, like so many other nuggets of scripture, I am curious to see if this verse might be intended for other purposes that can propel us forward in this life that, at times, feels like we are constantly being held down by invisible anchors with ropes that have tugged on our hearts for far too long.

I have walked through most of my life as an open target. I've allowed the arrows of words to hurt, to penetrate. I've allowed the actions of others to inform my character to such a point that I started to believe I wasn't worth anything good and, worse, worthy of love. I was quiet prey. I never let my captors know the depth of wounding that was taking place. I took it. I wallowed in it, and my cells ate it up like wildfire. I started to embody distrust in every human who crossed my path. My armor of protection was multi-layered, and my intuition grew stronger while my self-esteem waned.

When given a second lease on life, you evaluate every crevice of your soul. For me, trusting others still ends up being a valley miles deep. And I'm still stuck down there, but not as deep. I'm slowly making my way out. I see the light ahead, and it feels so good. With each truth I speak, healing takes place. And my body, your body needs this. It wants to be honored and seen as a vessel worth caring for.

People are going to make mistakes. They are going to hurt you. This is all part of navigating relationships. To meet someone who will stay even on your playing field is likely impossible. The hiccups we experience in relationships, especially those closest to us, often end up benefiting us in the end. There is a newfound sense of understanding one another, humbling ourselves, and growing closer. I know this isn't true for every encounter. The ones where hurt can leave a big wound; it's better to "detach" and pour into yourself to begin the mending process.

Before my diagnosis, I kept my biggest feelings in the smallest boxes. People often made me angry and took advantage of me for their benefit. I swallowed it. Once again, I am trying to be the "good Christian girl." *Love and forgive, love and forgive, love and forgive"* played on repeat in my conditioned 7-year-old mind. This is undoubtedly a vital truth to follow, but when all that loving and forgiving is poured out to others for their actions, you are slowly deteriorating the reserves of love you have for yourself. So now, when I feel challenged by a friend or family member who has hurt me and caused me to feel things that don't feel healthy, I take a very active approach. It's simple. "Let's talk about it." Most people immediately react. This is a natural defense mechanism. Remember, we are humans and are designed to self-protect. Their immediate reaction, especially if it is adverse, is not about you. This is them and a result of what they have to work through. And in the truth-telling exchange, your answers will come quickly. The answer is whether or not this person is honest, accepting, and, most importantly, one of your people. And understand that the Universe has a way of weeding out the energies that are not good for your being. But if you don't give the Universe space to work, it cannot work. The space is created through speaking. The space is created by unpacking small boxes of big emotions and subtle resentments.

What weighs you down emotionally will eventually weigh you down physically. A somatic response that, over time, can become chronic. Your body throws you energetic warning signals daily to keep you safe and healthy. But so many of us ignore these signals because we get so comfortable living in distress that we don't know what the alternative feels like. Trust me. It's like coming home when you can listen to your body and let the heavy stuff go. And once again, as much as I dislike the word "literally," it serves to be used well in this context. You begin to feel lighter. Joints feel better; backaches lessen; sleep is better; focus increases, and the list is endless. Your cellular self no longer has to expend energy feeding your "uncomfortable." It can pour into the more important stuff. For me, it was my blood. I had so many tiny boxes ready to explode and require maintenance that the most essential yet fundamental part of my body began disintegrating. My blood.

And possibly, the most crucial rule when truth-telling to another is the choice of words we use. And again, the bible does a better than adequate job of relaying the power of words. Scripture states, "The tongue can bring death or life; those who love to talk will reap consequences. Our words have the power to build people up and give them life or tear people down and bring them death. The words we speak can inspire and encourage others while, in the same sentence, deflate and encourage" (Proverbs 18:20). This is pretty straightforward advice, as well as the consequences of "building up or tearing down."

Let's be builders through our truth-telling. Someone has wronged you? Approach them with love and create a space of acceptance. You might be rolling your eyes right now. I get it. I've been there and am there a lot. But here's the thing... when you start seeing people through the lens of understanding who they are based on emotional baggage, you can better accept them for who they are. Again, their response to your truth-telling, especially if visceral or reactive, is not because of you. And when you do tell your truth, it is essential to stand in it. Stay grounded. Feel the earth beneath your feet. This gives you power and a sense of being in your body. The kickback for your body when you are mindfully aware of your power is magnificent. I picture my little cells having a party as they feel the nurturing I offer them.

And lastly, as you deliver your truth with a gentle tone, be sure to listen actively. Listen not only to their words, but also to their body language. Practice becoming an expert energy reader. You will be surprised how easy it is once you give yourself the freedom to be introspective about the person you are talking to. Affirm them for what they are feeling and sharing with you. This is so very important! People want to be seen, heard, and loved. When you practice these three principles in your conversations, you remove the heavy velvet curtain that keeps transparency off the stage. Over time, the most beautiful thing begins to happen. Instead of your relationships grabbing shields of protection whenever one of you feels threatened, the shields are placed down one at a time. You both feel more confident, trusting that you are now seen as a complete human, with flaws and all. You begin to teach each other how to dance in a relationship that is worth saving. Let people hurt you, but be mindful of how to respond. I've lost too many friendships because I retreated too soon. I didn't dare to be a truth-teller. Be the best builder around when it comes to your truth-telling.

Truth 24: Don't Get Stuck

If you continue actively reforming your thoughts, you will slowly back away from the "stuck" of who you think you are. In this case, you are limiting who you can become.

It's early June at the Jersey Shore—the traffic triples after Memorial Day. The boats bring welcomed energy. The air smells like salt, fish, and summer. For as much as some might think Jersey is "dirty." It's not. And that's all I have to say about that.

But with June comes July. And for me, July will never be the same month it was before 2022. I'm a month away from my diagnosis date, July 15th, 2022. This will mark my second anniversary. My body knows that the day is approaching. All the smells, the sun, the end of a school year, and the start of summer remind me that there was a point in life when I was slowly dying.

My brain feels so stuck. It's like I walk around with a bright orange Leukemia cancer flag tattooed on my forehead. I still feel like I have cancer, and I hate it. I hate that every time I see a commercial about cancer treatment, a pink ribbon, or a 5K awareness race, I go right back to "sick Sarah" mode. *Will it come back? How many years do I have left? Will the donor cells work long-term?* I'm an expert at creating mini-conversations in my brain that can multiply and send me into a tailspin of pretend sickness. And I know that the more I embody a lie or a truth, the more I will become it. And if I'm fully transparent, I haven't yet found the rest that comes with fully believing that I'm healed. I battle daily. I walk on the boardwalk, see hundreds of people on the beach, and wonder why they don't have

Leukemia. I see overweight individuals smoking and drinking daily, and wonder why they didn't get blood cancer. As I have said in previous pages, I would never wish this on anyone. I'll continue to take the approach of "Why not me?" So, I write this truth as a piece of healing for me. Maybe my words will encourage you and also help positively impact my recovery process.

I love to watch people. Study people. The body language, eye contact, or avoidance, and most importantly, energy. One thing I've found common among nearly everyone who has crossed my path is that we are all stuck on something in one way or another. That something might be regret for a mistake we made 25 years ago. Or a current situation that you feel defines you in such a way that you will never be the same again. And though that might be partly true, the other half is untrue. However, our brains tend to get stuck on the untrue. Our brains have an easier time attaching to the negative.

Think back to the details of what you consider the happiest day of your life. See how many of the details you can recall. The smell? The people involved? The setting? Now, switch gears and practice the same mindset on one of the most challenging, possibly trauma-informed days you have experienced. It is likely that the details and remembrances of this event have a sharper edge.

As you think about this event or this day, your heart rate will likely increase, you will feel a pit in your stomach, or there will be some other unexpected somatic reaction. This is because we embody the negative much more quickly than the positive. There is a more pronounced emotional response in the brain. But we can take action against the days, choices, mistakes, or diagnoses we find ourselves in that can rebuild our emotional health one cell at a time.

I like to think of stopping our thoughts of self-defeating and incriminating ideas as if it's a pause button on a TV remote. But this practice of pausing our racing thoughts does not come easily. Like many truths in this book, it's a practice. In my case, when I find myself going down the rabbit hole of more bone marrow biopsies in the future, I have to take an active approach of mentally listing all of the current positives related to the past 12 months of blood draws.

At least three times, I repeat to myself, *I am healthy, my donor cells are working, and I have had no bad news in 18 months*. And it works! I was surprised by how easy this was. It became clear to me one day. Wouldn't it be sad if, twenty years from now, I lived every day in fear that Leukemia would rear its ugly head? I have no crystal ball, but I have each day as its own.

And the most redeeming part of this practice is that it only leads to clearer thinking and less space for falsities to sneak in. If you continue actively reforming your thoughts, you will slowly back away from the "stuck" of who you think you are. In this case, you are limiting who you can become. When practicing active reversal of negative thoughts, your body celebrates you! It already knows who it wants you to be, but fear gets in the way. And fear, as mentioned in Truth 12, can be paralyzing. And paralyzation can get pretty comfortable if we live with it from day to day. And again, if I'm fully transparent, there are many days I'm paralyzed with the fear of being a single mom to five kids. Those falsities run through my brain as quickly as it takes to breathe one single breath.

Can I do this financially? What happens if the water heater breaks? Does my extended family still love me despite my choice against the laws of faith? What if I've ruined the lives of my children forever?

And it's in this millisecond of internal panic that I breathe deeper and visually imagine myself stepping away from my life to get a zoned-out view of how well I'm getting it done. I've learned to make five freezer meals on Sunday, pull them out when I get home from work, and pop them in the oven to attend lacrosse games and soccer games. I balance my budget every morning and earn extra money by working three part-time jobs in addition to my full-time job. I've learned that my God provides for me and doesn't shame me, and I no longer need to rely on accolades from Christians who feel safe in life, following the black-and-white rules. And it's in these moments of squeezing out of spaces too tight that my energy flourishes, and my cells celebrate. I'm getting it done well.

Be easy on yourself. This doesn't happen overnight. It's a daily practice of recognizing the habits of your thoughts. And it's as simple as that. It's a habitual way of thinking that gets comfortable for your brain. Daily affirmations taped on your bathroom mirror, car dashboard, and above the kitchen sink are an easy way to begin building up your internal power.

Don't get stuck on the choices you regret. Forgive yourself; you are human. Don't get stuck in your failures. Forgive yourself. You are human. Don't get stuck on repetitive thoughts that you're not enough. Love yourself. You are a beautiful human. Don't get stuck on the whys and hows. You are human. This is all normal, and working through life's process is like taking three steps up a mountain and then one step back. And though we may never reach the top, we are getting closer with every step, every breath, and every false truth.

November 2022: Walking Dead

I head into November with just a few weeks away from my admittance to Hackensack Medical Center for my transplant. I continue to wrap up testing, scans, and minor surgery to remove a nodule from my vocal cord. This is something entirely unrelated to cancer, but instead a direct result of overuse, as I had given over two hundred presentations during the previous school year. Another indicator that *I* was responsible for the breakdown of my health and overall well-being.

Since October served as a launchpad for irresponsible yet fun choices, I figured I might as well keep my streak going since everything to come wasn't guaranteed. I had difficulty holding onto my positive attitude and was tired of reading quotes and bible verses about strength. I let myself imagine the alternative of not coming home, the donor cells not working, and ultimately, what life would be like for my five children without their mother. I hated these thoughts and couldn't avoid them. They buzzed around my brain like a fly that wouldn't leave the room. And just when you think you're about to take down the fly, it buzzes off to a far corner, taunting you.

So, I give up and practice unhealthy avoidance. More bars, drinking, late nights, stupid decisions, and everything that comes with numbing my fear. And it wasn't so much a mindset of *I might not live* that had me walking the line. It had more to do with the anger, the why, and the uncertainty. And it all boiled down to "fuck you cancer," and watch me live without a fear of dying.

In hindsight, I don't regret the choices I made. I see it as all part of the process. It introduced a new sort of compassion for those who struggle with addiction as a means to escape. It advised me not to judge those who appear to be oblivious to the lifestyle choices they are making. The fact is, they *are* ignorant, and that's okay. Some day, they will be awakened and move through the recovery process, understanding that their choices, like mine, were a temporary solution to a problem too big to face. Pain is not measurable, but it's a pain, and it's their pain. They are allowed to make mistakes and learn from them. At times, consequences will follow, which is the unfortunate part of playing emotional roulette. But you are willing to play the game when pain runs deeper than one can measure.

It's November 8th, just six days away from the next big chapter. A routine checkup with my Leukemia doctor is what brings me here. Dr. F. opens the door and takes two quick steps in before she declares robustly, "The cells are in the country!" I recall Dr. R when he skated in to share the news of clean bone marrow scans with me. Both doctors shared the same enthusiasm, excitement, and unbridled emotion. Similar to receiving the Christmas gift an 8-year-old hopes for. It was a happy moment, a confirming moment, and the first moment that ensured all would move forward. I asked for a picture of Dr. F and me to document the moment, and I'm so glad I did.

It's November 14th. I sit in the passenger seat as Kyle drives the hour north to my new and temporary home for 21 days. We are silent. I can't figure out if it's in response to our current relationship status or because of the circumstances of the drive and the uncertainty of when or if I'll be making the drive back. Either way, he is here, and I feel safe. He knows me better than anyone, and I'm thankful he is beside me.

The hospital staff are waiting for me. I am greeted with smiles on the transplant floor. The smiles are genuine. I have passed the point of feeling like nurses and doctors are obligated to treat me like a human being. I go down the hall to my room and pass patients walking by me with machines in tow. There are many of them. All just walking, and I remember making a mental note that this all seemed strange. I let the image float by, anticipating that the chamber would become my home over the next three weeks. My room is basic; it feels like a yellow, synthetic space. It has all the hospital things.

Pink antibiotic hand soap, a handicapped chair next to the shower, a vinyl recliner, and a desk area. I place my bag on the bed and let out a sigh. I imagine that I'm an addict being admitted into isolated treatment for 30 days. It feels lonely, scary, and welcoming. I take a deep breath. I suggest Kyle leave as it's late, and the kids will want him to tuck them in. In reality, I just wanted to be alone because I needed to cry, and the best way to do that is when no one is around.

The following week is spent meeting new doctors, medical students, nurses, dietitians, chaplains, and social workers. I wonder if these people could ever comprehend how overwhelming these new meet-and-greets can be. It's similar to meeting your boyfriend's extended family for the first time. You're the newbie, and everyone else has these unspoken connections, and you can't make out who is putting on a smile for you and whose smile comes naturally. All of these strangers seem to want an emotional connection with me to trust them. The truth is. I've never trusted anyone—only myself. So, I stay guarded often. And I am well aware of my lifelong habit of pulling away when I feel threatened. I'm a turtle, have my shell, and tuck away in a hot second if I sniff lies, mistrust, manipulation, or judgment. This doesn't always work in my favor. I've snuffed out many potentially good relationships because of this flaw.

The first week of my 21-day stay involves intense preparation for the upcoming transplant. This involves hours and hours of chemotherapy, which means I stay in bed and wait for the hours to pass until I can get up. It also means blood draws at various times during the day and the night. I sleep through most of this process.

Unlike the purple poison, I'm barely phased by the milky- colored fluid dripping slowly into the tube attached to my catheter. Chemotherapy becomes a silent friend, and it comes in all different colors. It's there to give me hope, and I work as hard as possible to fulfill my end of the deal. Blood draws are constant, drugs are administered through my port that I don't know anything about, and the loneliness feels lonelier than the first stay. I figure this is because I'm farther from home, and FaceTime calls with my children make me feel like I'm in a different country. I don't answer FaceTime calls from my seven-year-old twins every evening because I don't have the energy to deal with the tears and the emotional thunderstorm that follows after the call. It's easier to take a Xanax and call it a day.

It has been reinforced several times since my admission that patients are to walk laps around the hospital floor daily. A large whiteboard with room numbers and dry-erase markers is near the nurse's station. It is here that we, the patients, record our laps. Being a competitive and overachieving person, I make a mental note to walk the most laps each day. I'm not tired during the first week of treatment. I walk 22 laps in the morning, 22 at 2 pm, and 22 at 5 pm. Totaling three miles a day for the first week. I'm proud of this and get compliments from doctors and nurses.

I often write the number 66 on the whiteboard and am usually in the lead. I feel as though the number 66 is indicative of the hell I'm about to endure with the upcoming transplant.

My machine comes in tow on these walks. His name is Hector. We became friends. He goes everywhere I go. We are constantly connected. I guide him as he walks beside me. When my right arm gets tired from holding the metal pole, I switch to my left arm. The other walkers give a slight nod as I pass. There are never words exchanged or friends made during these walks. As patients, we are too tired to deal with people and don't want to compare stories because theirs might be worse or better than ours.

Some walk briskly like I do, and their skin tone is natural. They are the newly admitted patients. Others walk slower and have yellowish skin. They wear slippers and want to finish this portion of their day. And then some walk with the aid of a nurse. They look gray and tired. There are bags under their eyes; they move slowly and step carefully to the side if I come up to lap them. These are the patients whom I might not see on tomorrow's walk. All of us are fighting to walk away from death. These walkers are walking into death, and they are aware of that. They cling to the nurse and are thankful for a human connection during their final days.

My days are mapped out hour by hour. It's the only way of getting the days to pass. There are the meal hours, the yoga hours, the reading hours, the napping hours, the phone call hours, the writing hours, the shower and cleaning my room hours, and the walking hours. The TV hours are saved until 7 pm. No earlier. I refuse to be sucked into the mindless oblivion of Netflix for 21 days. The 4:00 hour is the hardest. It's too late to nap, too many walkers are in the hallway, and I'm too tired for yoga or reading. I set an alarm on my phone for 5:01 pm. This is the alarm to remind me to order dinner. If I don't place my order within a few minutes after 5:00, I will be put on hold for up to 20 minutes while waiting to complete my order. The same music and hospital announcements repeat every 30 seconds. I can recite those announcements perfectly to this day, and I cringe whenever I call the hospital for an appointment and am put on hold. My stomach clenches, my heart beats faster, my breath becomes more shallow, and the visuals flood, overlapping one another. The yellow room, the smells, the ginger ale, cranberry juice, the beeping, and the saline bags all return. And I am reminded that trauma is a feeling more than a memory.

My three-week stay is outlined on a calendar for my reference. It looks like the calendar my mom had hung in her kitchen while I was growing up. This calendar is basic. There are no pictures; instead, there are boxes for each day of the month. I picture my mother's handwriting done in pencil for erasing. Her handwriting is as sweet as she is. It's her handwriting; I know I will miss it someday when I no longer receive her birthday cards that always start with "Dear Sarah Liz."

The difference is that my hospital calendar is flooded with codes, treatments, and things I didn't understand. There weren't dentist appointments, family parties, or track meets on this one. I circle November 21st with a red pen. This is transplant day. The day the nurses and doctors lightly call my "new" birthday. On my walks, I pass dollar store balloons strung to several hospital room doors. They are the nurses' way of bringing the slightest joy to patients, reminding them that transplant day marks a new beginning rather than the end.

November 21st arrives.

The side effects of chemotherapy haven't fully kicked in. I'm told I will start feeling the effects in a few days. Doctors stress that I should continue using my mouth rinse to prevent mouth sores from developing. I'm diligent with this—every hour. I'm confident that I won't be affected by this side effect. I usually shower at 6 pm, but my nurse wants me to take it early today. She said I'll be too tired to take it later. I'm confused, but I do what she wants me to. I still have my hair and take my time washing it while I shower. I dress for the day and wear my favorite green V-neck terry cloth shirt. I want to feel pretty, and I want to look the transplant in the eye and dare it to dominate me with fear. To this day, that same green shirt hangs in my closet, but I have yet to wear it. Emotionally, I'm not there yet.

I'm told the cells are "across the street" and will be delivered shortly. I'm drugged up on Benadryl and take a three-minute video on my phone documenting my feelings in the moments leading up to it. No one has seen that video except me—the next person to see it will be my donor.

Two nurses enter the room wearing the typical blue vinyl scrubs that indicate a product or medicine is about to be administered, requiring complete sterilization. Numbers are read, and questions are answered. The bag of marrow cells is small. The color reminds me of the red liquid left in the styrofoam tray once you take a steak out to grill. The nurse asked if I would like to hold the bag. It is the standard practice, a moment where I can look, connect, and barely comprehend what this one-pound bag of liquid represents. I've thought long and hard about whether or not I wanted a photo to document this moment. Until now, I had been determined not to take a photo because I wanted the mental picture to be my own. But then I remembered that there was another human who might have appreciated this photo. A nameless stranger somewhere in the world who was about to save my life. Green shirt, bag of cells, swollen eyes, and thinning hair. Good picture.

The procedure is pretty uneventful. I sleep, and my nurse stays in the room with me for the 45 minutes the cells are administered through my catheter. Mission complete, I continue to sleep. A few hours later, I tell the nurse through a daze that I will walk. She abruptly replies, "Not today, sweetie." I was not happy with her. How dare she instruct me on what to do?! Walking is healthy, and I have to keep my laps up. But mostly, I had this jaded thought that missing some laps one day might mean I would screw up the whole process. It's completely irrational, but this is the part of cancer that messes with your head.

What if I miss one of my meds? What if I don't drink enough water today? What if I'm some anomaly case the doctors have run out of answers for? What if the marrow doesn't work? What if I'm not eating enough protein? And what if I can't keep up the mental strength that has carried me this far? And could my mistakes cause the cancer to come back?

In hindsight, she told me not to walk because she knew I would be frustrated by my newly informed weakness. She knew that today's walk would not feel like the others. She knew I needed rest for tomorrow's walk and for just getting through tomorrow.

That night, I didn't sleep. I spiked a high fever, and I shook all over. My teeth chattered, causing my jaw to ache. I rocked back and forth, trying at the same time to keep the ice packs secure under my neck and on my forehead. I was helpless, and there was nothing I could do. My body is doing what it wants right now. Nurses flood in, all at the same time. I see navy scrubs all blurred together and all doing different jobs. One stands at my side. I hear her voice, but can't make out her face.

Blood is being drawn frantically from my catheter. Vials of blood are taken in glass bottles and transported to the laboratory. The bottles remind me of medicine that lined an apothecary shop in the 50s. Nothing feels right. It all feels wrong. I'm covered in heavy blankets, my head is pounding, and I strain my neck as I try to manage the chattering teeth that I have no control over. I moan. I squeeze my nurse's hand, and I realize that this is the beginning of my physical rebirth.

The days to follow feel like I'm trying to make friends with a stranger. Nothing feels the same. Every day, a new symptom presents itself. There's the bone aches in my jaw. A pain that replicates a toothache that can't be controlled by oxycodone. It's funny how against pain meds I was before cancer. I anxiously count down every 30 minutes until I have another dose to take the edge off, and that's all it does. Take the edge off. I sit in my vinyl recliner, icepack on my jaw, and try to distract myself with a Giants game I watch. I mainly focus on the fans.

They are just a few miles from my hospital room, and I can see the MetLife Stadium lights from where I sit. I'm angry with these strangers. They have done nothing to me except remind me that life is still happening out there, and it doesn't appear that any of them are dealing with bone aches.

Then there is the weakness. I give myself a pep talk to get up and out of bed to walk to the bathroom that might as well be a mile away. Nurses want to help me and make sure I don't fall. I refuse— every single time. My pride is too thick, and if I accept help, then that means that cancer is winning. Again, "fuck you, cancer, you're not taking away my dignity too." Walks are not the same. I now fall into a different category of walkers. My skin tone is yellowish; I have dark circles under my eyes, and I tend to look down.

I plug in my AirPods and listen to nothing. I want them there as a shield. If someone says "hi," I can ignore them, and they can chalk it up to me not hearing them. I'm not in the mood for small talk, and I'm annoyed at the nurses who talk about new restaurants they've tried and gel manicures they weren't happy with.

My walks go from 22 laps to 3-5. They are exhausting. I'm pissed. I can't make my legs go anymore. I grip Hector's cold, metal neck tightly and hold back tears. I want to rip out this machine and throw it through the picture window I've passed hundreds of times. I don't even look out that window anymore on my walks. It's just a reminder of regular life.

People are doing all the people-ly things. Cars running red lights, people on their phones as they walk across the street, and the constant continuation of lives that have no idea the hell that another human is having to fight just a block away. I hate them, and I don't even know them. I'm done with compassion. I walk with anger and hate.

And that's okay.

The mouth sores are next. Until now, I figured my hourly rinses would stave off the tiniest sores. I am wrong. I wake up one morning, and it hurts to swallow. I sprinkle honey and mix in bananas into my cream of wheat. I like my breakfasts and find them comforting. They are always the same. The hospital bread is tough and cheap. Eggs remind me of the homemade slime my kids make. The only fruits allowed are bananas and oranges because they are in their peels. Fruits and vegetables without their peels could bring deadly germs into my body.

I take the first bite of my breakfast and immediately cough it up. Cream of wheat and a partially chewed banana are now splattered all over the tray before me. It feels like razor blades are aligning my esophagus. I tried again without the banana. I can't do it. I try a sip of coffee. That makes things worse. I push the tray away. I start to cry.

There are limited moments of comfort when you're in a hospital as long as I was. You have to decide which moments are comforting and then enjoy them. Breakfast was a comfort; now, even that has been stripped from me.

It's time for morning meds, and I'm hungry. My nurse sees my pain and brings me a nasty liquid shot to drink down quickly before taking my meds. It numbs my throat for three minutes so I can get down the tiniest of pills. It turns into a long process of swallowing a few and re-trying over and over again on the larger pills. My meals are now raspberry sorbet, but it has to be mostly melted to get down.

Over the next four days, the mouth sores only get worse. I have a suction tube next to my bed that's sole purpose is to suck out the blood from my mouth. I use it every ten minutes or so. I take this all in stride. My nurse says it will pass in four days, and I believe her because these nurses have done this long enough to know exactly when the symptoms will begin and end. So far, they have maintained a perfect track record.

I am told that hair loss will occur on day ten after my chemotherapy treatment. A fleeting part of me thinks I will be the 0.5% of patients who won't experience hair loss. Another part of me wants it gone to prove to cancer that I don't give a fuck. Either way, I was afraid of losing my hair, not because of vanity but rather because of the emotional reminder that would be present every time I looked in a mirror. There are the subtle aches and deep pains of cancer that those who have not walked this road will never feel.

It's day 10 post-chemotherapy. I push myself up to a seated position on my bed as my custodian friend comes in to clean my floors. He saved my room for last on his rounds so that I could sleep until 8 am. We exchange positive affirmations and discuss the weather, as well as other random topics. Except this particular morning, things were different.

My white pillow is covered with endless amounts of hair. Clumps and piles all squished together. Some float to the floor, spread randomly across my sheets, and stick to my neck and chest. Its energy was mocking and rude. It didn't look like my hair. It looked like a monster that was proud I was emotionally succumbing to its tentacles. I started to cry a little.

My friend sees me. He doesn't say anything. Instead, he smiled tenderly and put a hand on my shoulder. He leaves the room when he is done cleaning, and my nurse then arrives. I'm sure he shared with her my unexpected and much-anticipated nightmare. She is Haitian and kind. But she is to the point; you would think she was rude if you didn't know her. She looks at me and stoically says, "It's time." This means that it's time to shave my hair.

My best friend arrived a few hours later. I only want her to be there for this. She offers to take a video. I abruptly snap at her and say, "No." Later, I apologize. The razor buzzes quietly, and my nurse takes her time for every stroke. She hums while she shaves my head. It's clear she has performed this routine hundreds of times, but not once do I feel a lack of empathy from her. My brain does what it always does. It imagines.

So, I imagine participating in some Hindu ritual or offering to the Gods. I half-smile to myself because I like how I think. The nurse is swift to pick up my hair. She has enough experience to know that seeing piles and piles of beauty that cancer has stripped is just too much for some patients. I walk to the bathroom. I look in the mirror, and what I see and feel shocks me. I see a beautiful woman. I see my cheekbones. I see my eyes. I see a powerful woman who is damned to win this battle even if she doesn't have a crown.

Thanksgiving Day arrives, and I try to resist checking social media throughout the day. The pumpkin pies, cozy family-filled living rooms, toasts, and golden turkeys. All of the simple things I now will never take for granted. At 4:00, the nursing staff announces that

186

there will be a Thanksgiving Day parade through the halls of the transplant floor.

As patients, we wait in anticipation at our room doors. Hector stands next to me as the other Hectors do with their masters. I smile inside because it's the saddest yet sweetest version of the Macy's Day Parade I've ever seen, but it is so powerfully informed by love.

The parade consists of multiple dollar store character balloons. It dawns on me that one of the nurses left her house 20 minutes early before coming to her shift to pick up the balloons. Mickey Mouse, Darth Vader, Sponge Bob, and Santa! A hospital bed is decorated with lights, tissue paper, and garland to replicate a float. The parade stops at every "home" (our rooms) and offers us a choice of champagne, red, or white sparkling grape juice. I am flooded with gratitude, and for the slightest of moments, I feel completely cancer-free. There is laughter and clapping on the floor. There is life. And that's all any of us are shooting for in the end.

It's November 30th, my oldest daughter's birthday. I was anticipating this day for my entire hospital stay. I have never not been with one of my children on their birthday. And out of all my children, even though she is the tough-on-the-outside type, her heart is tender, and I knew she would miss me. My Mollygrace Rose turns 16. The birthday all little girls imagine includes pink and sparkly things, heels, a cute dress, dinner out, a party, and, in a perfect world, a white jeep in the driveway with a bow on top. It is mostly wishful thinking for some teens and others, a reality.

My Molly didn't have a big celebration that day. I had a friend deliver her favorite red velvet cake. My dad picked up fancy cookies from her favorite spot. I hid her gift at the top of my closet and told

187

her where to find it. I left all the things that "look" like a birthday, but come nowhere near feeling like a birthday. That was the hardest day of November for me, and I'm sure it was much harder for her.

Truth 25: Manifest that Shit

Challenge yourself to practice tiny steps toward manifesting what you want and know you deserve.

I firmly believe that the Bible contains tender, applicable, and supportive truths that can hold and guide us through the beauty and despair of this life. In Matthew's book, I find a correlation between our power of manifestation and the truths of our lives. When awakened and embraced, this power within us allows the gifts to float to us.

"Ask, and it will be given to you; seek, and you will find; knock, and the door will be opened. (8) For everyone who asks receives; the one who seeks finds; and to the one who knocks, the door will be opened" (Matthew 7 7-8)

What does it mean to seek something? It's looking for that thing in unsuspected places. It's daily energy to find what you are looking for or may not. Seeking means putting forth effort toward what you need in the immediate or long term. To knock means for someone to open a door. Doors represent new beginnings, new life, light, transition, and moving forward.

As mentioned, we are excellent at getting in our way. The phrase "getting in our heads" can be applied here. But this verse gives us hope that we are worthy to receive. I always thought that the words sounded too simple. Ask and receive, seek and find, knock, and the door will open? The text sounded simple because I never put the words into action. I read the words for what they were. Just words.

189

But applying these words to the context of life could translate to the power that God has given us to manifest.

Faith is believing what we cannot see. And in many ways, manifesting works similarly. The difference is that manifestation requires a clear vision to be set forth. Faith is more concrete. It's a mindset shift applied to situations as they arise. Manifesting requires constant positive thoughts, all of which move toward a great outcome.

You give thought power to something you want to see come to light. When combined, the words "to manifest" might evoke a slightly esoteric vibe. We might ask ourselves what it means to direct our thought life to something we want. It seems too simple. But the key is understanding that the energy moving through you needs portals for release. And your cellular self is screaming for you to do great things. But if you don't feed your cells with daily mental pep talks, the Universe will have nothing to work with.

Your vibrations have the power to attract what it is you want. And since most of us don't live in this state of belief, we find ourselves dreaming big dreams and keeping it just to that. Just dreaming. But to manifest something is a call to action. It's writing goals on Post-it notes around your home. It's working on something a little bit each week or each day that you want to see grow. But the most powerful tool you have in your wheelhouse is your mind. Let your imagination take you to the biggest and brightest movie scene of what you want to see blossom.

I write this book mainly for my children. I want them to understand my heart, my faults, my mistakes, and my desires for them. I also find myself manifesting the hell out of these pages so that the readers will go far beyond the five I love the most in this world. I don't manifest these pages for fame or fortune. I manifest because I want to help others. I'm a helper, not a healer. But I want to teach people how to be their own healers. We all have the answers. They are right there, sitting beneath the fragile and thin layers of doubt and fear. I want others to understand that to live with joy, love, peace, and, most importantly, health, you must honor all of who you are.

The most remarkable aspect of the manifestation process is that it becomes intuitive with practice. You begin dreaming more, envisioning, and feel motivated and excited about what you believe will come to full completion someday. The more you practice, the more patient you become because you build tiny bits of confidence that the thing you are giving energy to will happen.

I've been divorced for 6 months and was separated 18 months prior. My twin nine-year-olds sleep on the floor in my room. They do this because their world was turned upside down two years ago when I was diagnosed. Then, their world was pulled inside out with the finality of divorce. They don't feel safe. There hasn't been much they can control. So they flood my room with pillows, blankets, and stuffed animals to create a nest of safety until they are strong enough to work through the messy feelings hiding under the covers.

But when my Charlie asks to snuggle with me, I love it for two reasons. The first reason is that I love being next to a heart that had once beat below my own for nine months. But secondly, I love having him next to me for those small moments because he's warm and close. I move him slowly back to his little nest once he's asleep, and miss the days when holding him felt squishy and squirmy.

191

I miss going to bed with someone. Sex is sex. That's in a different category. But being next to someone and intertwining energies in many ways is more powerful than a physical connection. And I want that someday. Kyle and I didn't have that.

My standards are high for a future partner. On paper, my standards look ridiculous and taunt me into thinking I'll be single for the rest of my life. But this is where I manifest. I see myself in a relationship someday where the other person understands me better than I do, where that person sees my ugly stuff as more beautiful than the physical stuff. Where the room shifts when we walk in together. I'm the last piece to his puzzle, and he's the last piece to mine.

It will happen, I am confident. I am not seeking. I fully surrender to the ways of this world and the magic that can happen when I take my hands off the wheel.

Challenge yourself to practice tiny steps toward manifesting what you want and know you deserve. Nothing is too big or outlandish. It all starts with morsels of thoughts, then snapshots in your brain of beautiful pictures of what you already know is waiting for you. Eventually, you start believing this thing or idea will happen, and it starts to happen because, without being fully invested, you are already investing with your thoughts. When we think about something long enough, especially if it's positive enough, our bodies and brains can't help but start navigating our choices and decisions to support our manifestations.

Scripture nailed this truth: "Ask, and it will be given to you; seek, and you will find; knock, and the door will be opened." Each piece of this trifecta of wisdom informs us that we have the power, no one else. We are the ones who are given complete allegiance to set forth what it is we want. And God, the Universe, wants to provide you with good things. He wants to give you these things because you are his child. You are created in His image, and He wants to see us living in joy and abundance.

I'm standing in front of an audience at a small bookshop, reading the forward to my book. I'm sitting in a plush pink chair in a local theater, discussing my book, ideas, and inspirations. My kids are part of the crowd. I'm on a plane and traveling to give a book talk somewhere. I'm invited to speak on podcasts. I'm signing books at Barnes & Noble in New York City. I'm in a parking lot leaving a gig and see a 23-year-old girl crying in her car. She sees me; she steps out. She said she was waiting for me to walk out of the venue. She says, "Don't worry, I won't tell you my problems. I need to hug you. I need to feel your power because you just helped me to step into my own." I manifest all these moments daily, but the one I look forward to the most is the last.

Truth 26: Ask For Help

You are the author and sculptor of your life's work. However, to perform your best work, you must step into the world and allow others to help you along the way.

I grew up on a farm. As a kid, I always followed this statement with an explanation that it was a "clean farm." I was afraid to be considered the farm kid who might be caught smelling like manure. There were always a few of them in a graduating class, as we lived in an area where farms were part of the land.

I hold gratitude for my childhood experience. Miles and miles of trails where I rode my beloved horses, and where getting lost on a snowmobile meant walking to a stranger's house, asking for directions. A concept that today's youth will never get to experience, due to the devices in their hands that provide a lifeline and answers to all the world's questions. Hideouts in pine trees where forts were made and where our mom's kitchen pans ended up. My neighbor friends justified our "borrowing" as we needed supplies for our pretend kitchen to make mudpies and soup out of stinkweed.

Memories are plenty and endless. The greatest gift growing up on a farm gave me was the realization that work is an integral part of life and that when we work hard, we achieve good results. I became an expert at cleaning out horse stalls once a week. I looked forward to laying down fresh bedding for my horse. It felt like wrapping a baby in the softest blanket. This was a good result. My siblings, my parents, and I each had our riding lawn mowers and sections of lawn for which we were responsible. My sister was better at making nice, neat lines in the lawn. And I remember comparing her results with mine. These were good results of hard work. Weeding, vacuuming out the pool, throwing and bailing hay, and laying mulch were tasks I was assigned to do, and through rolled eyes, I did them.

My parents prided themselves on taking care of a 70-acre plot of land by themselves and with the help of my siblings, myself, and the boyfriends I dated. Rarely did they ask for help. My dad never wanted to hire anyone to do the lawns, and all the fixing of machinery that consistently broke was for him to figure out. And he always did. He will always be the most intelligent man I know.

However, pride got in the way of all this work. I don't think my parents or I knowingly put our foot down to do things independently. I think it's more of a habitual way of living that we find ourselves in. And the longer we hold onto habits, the more they define us.

I fell into this way of living for 44 years. I insisted on doing things on my own for two reasons. The first reason was self-sabotage. I wanted to prove to myself that I was strong enough not to ask for help. The second reason was to prove to others that I was strong enough not to ask for help. Both reasons were born out of pride and the unhealthy standards I had put on myself.

And the backward part of all of this was that I started resenting people. *Why are they not helping me? They must be selfish.*

Upon reflection, this was not the case at all! I was giving off the energy that I could do things on my own. I've learned post-cancer that someone else will always do it. Whatever that "it " is, there is always someone else who will carry part or all of the burden. And when practiced enough, you begin to feel empowered. You start to stand in the truth of giving your precious time to the things that are healing for your body.

It took me a while to feel comfortable asking for help. It was hard at first. Thoughts like:

Am I putting this person out?

What if they are saying yes out of obligation?

What if they didn't mean their offer?

This is old Sarah's way of thinking. My cellular self had grown so accustomed to giving that receiving felt foreign and uncomfortable. I discovered through my sickness that people want to help. They heard of my diagnosis and flooded my GoFundMe with donations in just a few days. I felt guilty. They took my kids back to school shopping while I was in the hospital. I felt guilty. My parents and in-laws drove hours weekly to come down and help with the kids. I felt guilty. My school and community provided me with months of nightly meals, served every day at 5 pm. I felt guilty. People flooded my hospital room with gifts, lotions, and books that would help pass the time. I felt guilty. And I hated being in the position where I wasn't the helper but the one being helped.

Yet, through the process, I was humbled into a corner of what I like to call "healing through helplessness." It took time to get used to my new role. Yet once I bowed to the gifts and services I was offered, my body took deeper breaths, and I found relief knowing that my kids were cared for in every possible way. People want to help because that's how we were designed.

I have always compared this way of technological living to the human connection hundreds of years ago. I picture a village of children running barefoot, laughing, and playing with anything they can find. I see groups of females gathered at tables, weaving cloth or around a fire, preparing a meal for their tribe. The men work together on building and hunting. And in this picture, the common theme is helping. This machine runs efficiently, as no additional machines are needed, because everyone involved is contributing.

There is no resentment, equal distribution, and a goal in mind with each task. That's how we were designed. As humans, we need help. This life doesn't come with a rulebook, and it prides itself on throwing the most unexpected curveballs when they are least expected. We must realize that we are giving each other a gift when we put aside our control tendencies and soften to the helpers on deck.

We need to stop working harder than our bodies can handle. We devise excuses to justify our need to over-commit and constantly do things ourselves out of pride. I can fully attest that once you loosen the reins, you not only find physical rest but also begin to dive into the "whys" of not asking for help. Or the "whys" of overworking. Were you avoiding something too dark to look at? Were you hiding from something that you didn't want to come to terms with? Our bodies have a clever way of defending against what is too much to bear emotionally. For me, it was my marriage.

If I had asked for help and not tried to do it all alone, I might have lessened the emotional feeling of defeat that was sucking me dry. If I worked four jobs without a moment to come up for air, I could cleverly avoid moments of stillness to reflect on my unhappiness.

197

That moment of silence didn't come until July 15, 2022, when I sat helpless in a hospital bed just moments after my doctor shared that my body contained one of the most lethal cancers out there. My body gave up. Every helpless cell waved a white flag of surrender. And I had no choice but to fall flat on my face and give in, and then begin the process of learning to listen.

You are the author and sculptor of your life's work. However, to perform your best work, you must step into the world and allow others to help you along the way. Since God made us in His image and, in addition, gifted us uniquely, doesn't it make sense that we can accomplish great things with and for one another? Put pride aside. Walk yourself to the cozy corner of humility. Get quiet and learn how powerful it is to say yes to the helpers. Because when you say yes to the helpers, you are saying yes to yourself.

Truth 27: Do The Scary

Life will test you, but it will always catch you.

Tomorrow, I will say goodbye to my first kindergarten class. With them, over the past 180 days, I have felt loved. With them, I felt complete. Without them, it would be a hard feeling to get used to.

Five hours after final hugs and tear-filled eyes with 16 6-year-olds, I will board a plane with my most precious cargo. I've been a saver my whole life. An attribute my dad instilled in me, and I'm glad he did. Kyle and I didn't go on lavish vacations and rarely took the kids to dinner. I regret that now. But tomorrow, I'm going to change that, and I'm scared to be doing this alone. I have my itinerary and all receipts neatly organized, yet I feel like I'm walking into this 6-day adventure with a blindfold over my eyes. Swinging at the piñata of magical Orlando in hopes of a jackpot of memories, not treats, will fall into my children's laps.

I'm going on this trip for lots of reasons. I have one year left with my beautiful, powerful, yet soft oldest girl. How did playing with dollhouses and having tea parties turn into visits with her boyfriend over time with me? Secondly, I make this trip to celebrate the strength my kids have displayed throughout these past two years of hell. They deserve it. Lastly, I do this trip because I can. Not because I can afford it. Instead, because I'm healthy, and I'm here, and I'm a survivor. The list of "ands" is endless in my mind. And though I'm scared, I'm diving anyway.

Kids think the word scary means monsters under the bed and dark corners in the room. Adults think of scary as losing a job, ending relationships, and starting new ones. A lot of life occurs between childhood and adulthood, and we organically shift our embodiment of the word "scary" to label things unique to our way of living. But the scary I'm referring to here is the kind that rattles who we are and what we think we might be capable of doing. A railroad is straight, smooth, and predictable until it's not. As Robert Frost's infamous poem quotes, "Two roads diverged in a wood, and I– I took the one less traveled by, And that has made all the difference." You see where I'm going here. If we stay on the same track, we are essentially staying still. We become stagnant in realizing our full growth potential. And the more we rot in the normalcy of life, the more blinded we become to our power.

We must face the scary parts of life to prove our mastery over self-doubt and screaming insecurities. We must feel our hearts racing with fear and trepidation to reap the rewards that could land us in the land less conquered—a land that could bring far more joy than we could have ever imagined.

I realize I'm applying this principle to preparing for a six-day family vacation with kids in tow. This seems like a simple endeavor, but for me, it's not. I haven't flown in 10 years and am the sole adult responsible for my children. I'm trusting that all of this goes as "planned." And other than a few reservations, I have no plan. And that's the scary part.

We have to look at our lives like a four-semester report card. Yes, it's a cheesy teacher reference. The result is mastery, yet for most of us, the task at hand or the scary thing we are challenging ourselves to step into is often referred to as "needs improvement." When facing the scary, I am in life's "progressing" stage. Leukemia and a divorce were certainly fear-filled, with questions I didn't have answers for. And considering my Type A, all-boxes-checked personality. Let's say this didn't go too well with how I'm wired. However, it all worked out somehow.

Life will test you, but it will always catch you. I'm confident of that. But that's where the word scary comes in: to test and support you. As referenced in "Fear Has No Power," I apply the same principle here. Do the things that scare the hell out of you. You want to do them. Your body wants to do them. Your mind wants to do them, and the Universe wants to celebrate you. After it celebrates you, it wants to use you to do more scary things, giving you opportunities you could have never come up with on your own.

Stop trying to do things on your own. Stop hopping on the trains of life that lead you to one scripted destination you know you will get to without hiccups. I believe Mr. Frost's poem is so embraced because it penetrates all of us, yet most of us don't live by it. His message sounds nice in a poem; it looks nice in our imagination, but it's too scary to apply on a daily basis.

Sitting in the quiet takes a few moments to ask your body what it needs to flourish. Is it to change careers? Go back to school? Come out to your parents? Leave a relationship? Face addiction and get help? What is the scariest thing in life that holds you back from what you know is there? And that whispering knowing is your full potential. I ask myself, what if I put my entire life out there for my family or the world to see through written text, and the only thing that comes of it is judgment? But what if it doesn't? What if I reach a point in life where I am fully supported in what I was called to do? This is scary.

And understand that you don't have to take the first step into these scary endeavors alone. Be vulnerable to those around you, ask for support, and ask them to listen. Not to offer advice but instead to listen. They might come off to you as if they are the stronger ones. They are not. They have their list of untouchable fears, too, but they are not yet where they can imagine taking the first step. The full circle reward in this process is that, by example, you are permitting others to do the same.

Ten years ago, I knew my marriage was over, but I was determined to save it in any way I could. I planned vacations for just Kyle and me, made dinner reservations, and tried to extend his time in the studio creating paintings. But after a few years of feeling defeated, my therapist suggested that divorce might be the answer. My initial response was a heel dug deep into the ground of biblical laws and expectations. First, it's a sin. Second, I will have zero support from my family. And third, I will demolish the future for my children. As most things do with time, my views softened, and I started to feel the gentle hand of the Universe on my back, nudging me forward with affirmations of support.

My dear cousin, with whom I share boatloads of childhood memories, had decided to end her marriage just two years before mine. When I heard the news, something within me shifted. It was as if a switch had been turned on. My internal language went like this: *She's divorced. She did it. Our entire family still loves her. She's so brave. She's so incredibly brave. And she's still loved. And maybe*

I, too, will still be loved. So, I leaned on my cousin for support. I asked every possible question I could.

Most importantly, I wanted to know how she and her body felt. She supported me. I was the older cousin and the one she looked up to. She was now the one holding space for me. Support for one another's scary decisions of self-empowerment doesn't have to come through close family members. Life puts people in your path who can support your growth on a day-to-day basis.

Find a quiet place where you feel safe. Ask yourself what you need to step into that you don't feel ready for yet. You will get the answer immediately. The Universe waits outside a door for you to open at all times. It's quiet and patient, but can't open that door for you unless you unveil your whole self. You will take a tiny step through that door and want to retract immediately.

This is normal. This is the human brain, not the spirit part of you. Don't step back. Instead, breathe and stay in that tiny place as long as needed. Through your breath and stillness, you will gain strength. And once you take that second step and tiny blessings start to sprout, you can't wait to see where the following steps will take. Being scared is good. If you weren't scared, you wouldn't know how to overcome anything and create space for new and better things.

Truth 28: What Lights You Up?

What lights you up? What penetrates your soul so that you want to do it when you think about it?

I grew up riding horses. Competitively at times, and other times, silence and nature smell through the winding trails of my 70-acre property. As a 17-year-old, I knew not to take this for granted. This property wasn't something any of my friends had. So, I relished the rides, the serenity, and the place where I started learning how to think. Riding to me was more than sitting on the back of a powerful animal. It was solace. I felt safe. Somehow, the two of us blended to be one.

Reflecting on my riding, I realize that so much of it was intuitive. When I overthought the course, the horse responded with subtle reactions of obstinance. When I let go of the reins (so to speak), the horse glided over jumps and switched leads effortlessly. I miss those days. I miss my dark, sassy Thoroughbred, who didn't cut the race track. But he made the cut for me. I miss the quarter horse, who was looked down upon in the show ring because she turned her hind leg in her gate. She didn't cut it as a barrel racer or an English show stopper, but she was my everything. Both horses were slightly off in their identity, so I connected with them. I have always felt a little bit off with mine. We understood each other. We had something in common.

I loved riding because it made me feel powerful. I knew I belonged in the saddle, where no one could tell me how to do things. I was the one who knew—no one else. And the bond between those animals and me was something special. I still remember how warm and soft the necks of those horses felt as they stood still as statues, absorbing my tears. Those silly teenage tears that were usually in response to a high school boyfriend. But so still those beasts stood. They knew that they needed to hold space for me. That was a big part of their job. Riding to me was everything. Running was nothing. Running was like the distant cousin that wanted to connect with me. So, I connected because I felt obligated. That cousin took its place. There's no doubt. But I wonder where my first love would have taken me.

Many times, I Google search for local riding barns in my area. For whatever reason, I'm never brave enough to email the venue or attend a lesson. I feel so far detached from that time in my life. Yet underneath the layers of the past 25 years, the smells in the field, the four-count beat of post-ups still reside. The exhilarating feeling of hurling over a double Oxford is embedded in my sensory DNA. And I wonder if I could do that again. This lights me up. Thinking about it is one thing. Doing it is another. And this takes bravery at my age. I'm 46, and I ache every morning. I take 10 minutes to stretch out my lower back, neck, and feet. I used to roll my eyes at aunts and uncles who would complain and compare notes about such things at family gatherings. I get it now. The body is designed to function for a certain amount of time. And I don't have much time left to participate physically in the things I love doing.

Like I do with most things, I wonder why we don't make time or space for the things that make us happy. Is it the roles we play in this world that we feel attached to? Is it a lack of time? There's always more time in any day. It's just how you decide to divvy it out. People do what they want to do. Is it complacency, getting stuck in the Ground-Hog Day-like motions of life? I'm assuming it's a blend of all of those reasons.

When presenting hundreds of self-care and restorative practice workshops to educators before I fell ill, I would ask them to remember who they were in their early twenties. Some would laugh and reference drinking their way through that period. Others were quiet and looked at me. Even though they were looking at me, their minds were elsewhere. Happy places. A land that they missed and knew pieces of it were still available if they dared to put themselves first. I didn't expect them to leave and start painting classes or dive into swimming again. I just wanted to plant a seed of thought that maybe one person would discover this, and it would make all the difference in their day-to-day living.

I think it's essential to occasionally evaluate how much you are giving or honoring yourself. This isn't about getting massages, pedicures, or a new suit or dress. This is about giving to the true you, the one who is desperate to be remembered and honored.

As I've referenced many times and will continue to, all you've to do is spend a few hours with five-year-olds playing on their own. It's fascinating to watch that they need no gadgets, devices, or playgrounds to use their imagination. The subtle loss of imaginative play and washing my children's hair is something that disappears as if it's vapor, just whisked away. Children play according to their design. There are the leaders, the followers, and the ones who find their way quietly amidst the "let's pretend..." language of their peers. I bring this up because children know what they love and aren't afraid to explore it and feed that growing desire. But the older we become, the more we let peers, our world, or even our own families decide who we should be and what we should like. I've tried hard to make it clear to my children that it's time to let it go when something isn't giving them joy anymore. I believe this is a way to honor yourself. I want them to figure out what lights them up and excites them. With two teenage girls in the house right now, they would likely say shopping, but I'm hoping they will discover their passions and pursue these desires with as much energy as possible over the next few years.

My middle, Stella, is an outstanding soccer goalie. She found herself in the net by accident at the age of seven. Now, at 15, she hasn't played any other position on the field. I love watching her play. Her quiet and, at times, clumsy spirit off the field changes within a millisecond of her stepping on the turf. Her walk changes; she knows she's in charge, and the other team is sizing her up. I memorize her pregame rituals and believe it's the part of her brain she inherited from me.

She dives, leaps, comes out of the box, and tackles girls twice her size. She rarely complains about practices and sometimes rides her bike to a soccer field to practice goal kicks. Whenever she goes, I ask her, "Are you okay?" She looks at me and says, "Yeah, I'm just going to practice stuff," and off she struts with that confident, athletic gate, and I'm jealous. I'm jealous because I was never allowed to fully immerse myself in my passions the way I had wanted to.

I had a friend in high school whose locker was next to mine every year because our last names were just one letter apart. We weren't that close, but close enough to share secrets while spraying each other's bangs with Aqua Net hairspray and then looking in the tiny locker mirror to check that there were no pesky flyaways. Her school attendance was stellar, and she was always at her locker before me.

One morning, she wasn't, but I didn't think much of it. Soon after, the energy in the school changed. Something had shifted. Teachers walked by with red, puffy eyes, and the principal walked briskly into each classroom, privately speaking to each teacher individually. I was annoyed because I felt that, as a student body, we were being left in the dark about whatever tragedy had just taken place. And I knew it was something bad because I felt it. And that might have been the first time that energy informed me that bad news was coming.

My friend did not come to school that morning because she died in a fatal car accident. Students were let out mid-morning. My dad picked me up in his Verizon truck while on duty. On the way home, I looked out the window, trying to wrap my head around these unrecognized feelings. The only thing I could think about was getting home and saddling up my horse and riding fast, faster than my horse would want to go. And that's what I did. My parents didn't try to fix or talk to me; I was so grateful for that. They knew that I needed to do what I needed to do. I don't know how long I was out on those trails, but I know I was there a long time. I raced across the field fast enough to feel every strand of hair fall out of place. I didn't care about my perfectly sculpted bangs just hours prior; I wanted to feel a mess because that's how I felt inside. This is where I learned that our passions can care for us in the most awful moments.

Truth 29: Shit Happens, But It's All Redeemed

I've concluded that perspective plays a crucial role in helping us navigate these storms.

I watched her move with ease around the bar. Reaching for Tito's, Casamigos, and Hendricks without even looking down. She was the captain, and this was her bow. She was proud as she floated through the motions. I felt silly standing at the bar asking for three virgin strawberry daiquiris and a virgin pina colada.

I was a classic tourist whom she was forced to fake smile at and oblige as she had been trained to. I said, "Thanks so much; I know they're a pain to make. When you're done, I'll give you my drink order." She looked at me and winked, " Honey, I can multitask better than the best of them." Her confidence preceded her, and I loved that. We talk as most bartenders do when things aren't too busy.

I share my story; she absorbs it like a sponge absorbs water. She asks questions, and I feel apprehensive. I don't want to talk about cancer in such a way that it celebrates sickness. And that's how I feel sometimes. When I talk about cancer, it's always with one goal in mind. Encourage the listener to consider joining the bone marrow donor list, if their age allows.

She stops mid-shake of my margarita and says, "Baby, you have a story to tell, and it's a big one. I see you on podcasts and presenting to hundreds." I'm humbled and feel like a little kid who was just granted a gold star for not doing much.

I returned to my crew of four, who sat poolside, feeling like they were on a lavish vacation. I did my best to give them all the bells and whistles, least expensively and lavishly possible. I have also succeeded with an Airbnb and a clubhouse package. I was proud of myself. It starts to drizzle soft drops of heated Florida rain. The kids are done anyway. The teen girls are happy with their tan lines, and the 9-year-olds are whining. We packed, and I encouraged them to finish their drinks, which I had spent $70 on.

On my way out, I blew a kiss to my bartender friend. She shouts, "Hold on, baby, I need to hug you!" She hurries out, her patrons are annoyed, and she embraces me like a cousin I haven't seen in years. It was one of those hugs. Heart to heart, two humans, no names exchanged, but energy understood without words. She was someone who crossed my path and helped me move forward.

In some ways, I wish I had known her name. Yet, at the same time, I don't. Something about that three-second embrace informed me that she was weathering her storm. Without a chance to actively put words together, I say in her ear mid-embrace, "Remember this, shit is going to happen, but it's always redeemed." I think to myself, *damn girl, that's good*. I take note of the book material and make a mental note to store it in my phone's notes app when I get to the car.

We released from the hug. She looked at me, both hands on my shoulders, and said, "Take care of yourself, honey. I love you." Look at that —vulnerability in action. Two humans who are just being real; the result is as sweet as my mom's homemade strawberry rhubarb pie, crust and all.

211

And this is a truth we all know. Shit happens. This life is parallel to that of raising kids. When you think you're sailing through age two and mastering the potty training challenge, you reach age three, where Lord us with the power-yielding 30 lb. mini monsters. Or when you pat yourself on the back for your connection with your eleven-year-old. They talk freely about school drama and share their thoughts, laughing with you. And then, poof, just like that, you wake up one day to a twelve-year-old in your living room who might as well be a different human because you have no idea who this person is.

Life is smooth, but then it's not. And then it's smooth again, but you brace yourself for the subsequent trial or unexpected turn around the next corner. Cancer informed me that I'm no different from any other human. I worked out daily, ate healthy, and was a personal trainer and 500-hour yoga teacher trained in prenatal and children's yoga. My life was centered around health and fitness.

And then Leukemia. Right there for my eyes to read for the first time when my doctors handed me a paper from a fancy blood lab out west, I resented them for giving me this paper because it felt like they were trying to prove something. The image etched in my brain forever at the bottom of the medical document. In red, bold letters that fit well to deliver the blood cancer message: Conclusion: Acute Myeloid Leukemia with FLT3 mutation

We are all human, and though this life is a gift, it's also tough to navigate. I've concluded that perspective plays a crucial role in helping us navigate these storms. Bad things will happen, but it's how we decide to respond to them. If you feed a situation with negative thoughts and allow yourself to fester in them, that's all your brain will be trained to do. But the same principle applies here with the practice of anything you are trying to become better at. The more water you drink, the healthier you feel. The more five-year-olds practice riding a bike, the quicker they will master their first moving vehicle. The more you eliminate fast food, the better you will feel. The more you practice the guitar, the better a musician you will become. Practice doesn't make perfect, but practicing anything can improve it. And I think better delivers less pressure than perfect.

I said to Cancer from day one, "You picked the wrong human to mess with." I actively decided not to give this monster what it wanted from me emotionally. I refused to hide under the sheets of fear and self-loathing. I realized quickly that sulking in my diagnosis would go nowhere good. Long days isolated in a hospital room were beyond difficult, where often, the only thing I looked forward to was the next meal. Even this was questionable, depending on whether I could keep food down.

My character was tested, and the assessment tool was my internal dialogue. I also learned quickly to apply one question to each delivery of information from my doctor. The question was simple, but it helped my brain to turn shitty situations into redeeming ones. My doctor would present blood counts, bone marrow results, bone density results, and side effects for the upcoming chemotherapy treatment. I would ask myself, *What's good about this information/ situation?*

Instead of being scared of chemotherapy reactions, I decided to be grateful for the medical scientists who spent years developing a drug that was saving my life. Instead of fearing the following bone marrow biopsy procedure and the physical pain it held, I assured myself that I had a doctor who not only cared about the meticulous care it took to retrieve a bone sample but also my comfort as well. She never held back from asking how I was doing throughout the procedure and increased the numbing agents as needed. I would grip bed rails or the hands of nurses through these procedures and repeat affirmations over and over in my head. *I can do this. I am strong. It will be over soon. You've got this, Sarah. Just breathe.* These words held power, propelling these awful situations toward redeeming results.

I had a close friend visit me during treatment, and she asked me how I was doing. I appreciated this question because she wanted to hold space and give me a safe space to unload the heavy emotions jumbled together in one big mess. I thought about this question for a few moments. She was patient. And my response floated out of my mouth as if the words weren't ones I would have chosen. "Honestly... I'm thankful for cancer." She looked at me, head cocked, and questioned further. "Are you?"

And again, I was grateful for her challenging me emotionally. Not many friends know how to do that well. It's a delicate balance of loving an individual you care about and holding them accountable to a level of responsibility you hope they can handle. I looked at her and said with quiet confidence. "Yes, I am. I am." And upon reflection, my body answered her question because it was trained to.

I speak as much truth as possible to myself and continue to do so. And the umbrella of thought I will continue to cling to is this: bad things will happen, but they will always be used. But they will only be used if you allow them to be.

If I had not been given a life-threatening diagnosis, I don't think I would have left a marriage. If I had not been given a life-threatening diagnosis, I would have continued drinking nightly glasses of wine, overtraining at the gym, and getting five hours of sleep. If I had not been given a life-threatening diagnosis, I would still be saying yes to everything while living in resentment. Cancer taught me how precious I am. I am, you are, a rare jewel to be handled with care, kept safe, and admired. And I would much rather live a life where I view my life as a gift and not something to be taken for granted.

If I had not been given a life-threatening diagnosis, I would not have been given the chance to hug a nameless stranger at a Florida clubhouse bar. I would not have been able to connect energetically with someone who needed me as much as I needed her. This was a small but powerful gift. Cancer has given me big gifts and little gifts. And trust me, the smaller boxes with tiny bows often hold the most precious jewels.

Truth 30: Forgive

Forgiveness allows the heart of another to bow to yours with no wall in between.

To forgive someone might be one of the hardest things we are called to do in this life. It's not an instinct we were born with. It's something that most of us are taught to practice as children. A child steals a toy from another and is then prompted to say, "I forgive you." And perhaps some would disagree with the parenting practice I have implemented with my children and the students in my Kindergarten classroom. However, I think it's essential for children to learn at a young age that we are all imperfect, make mistakes, and disappoint one another. Practicing forgiveness brings growth and a deeper connection. Forgiveness allows the heart of another to bow to yours with no wall in between.

But as we move through life, walls start building themselves, and with time, those walls sink deeper into their foundations, becoming much harder to knock down or, even better, disintegrate. The longer we sink into resentment and refusal to forgive, the stronger those walls become. And before we know it, forgiving someone who has wronged you doesn't become an option because you've already decided it not to be. And what's unfortunate about this is that you are dis-servicing yourself. This might seem counterintuitive, but it's not.

It's straightforward. When you choose not to begin the process of forgiveness, you are feeding the anger. You are giving it fuel to grow, and over time, that growth becomes so big that the wall you

216

are creating between you and the other person seems too impossible to begin to chip away at. And this is where the word humble comes into play.

Often, being unable to forgive is related to pride. Humble takes a back seat to its cooler brother, pride. But the wiser of the two brothers is the younger one. Humble knows that good things will happen, and character will deepen when he practices his gift. Pride is built out of fear, and fear has no power. We must first self-assess and ask ourselves if pride is in the driver's seat or if the fear of forgiveness is rooted more profoundly than that. And maybe you're thinking that even the idea of forgiving someone who has hurt you immensely is not possible. And that's okay. You aren't there yet.

What I'm suggesting instead is that you imagine what it would look like and feel like if you were to start the process of forgiveness. This is a mental image that may never be put into practice. And again, that's okay. But dipping your toe into what forgiveness might feel like will translate to subtle ways of healing on a cellular level. Our body knows what it holds onto, but can't release these things unless we allow it.

Just as we are called to forgive others who have wronged us, we are also called to forgive ourselves. I've made many mistakes and choices that I'm not proud of. I will forever be transparent about this. When we dare to be transparent with one another, we invite others to do the same. And what's born from this is love and acceptance. And that's all anyone in this world wants. We want to be accepted and feel loved.

I am still learning how to forgive myself, but it's a challenging process. It's super hard. Ironically, forgiving myself is difficult, given that my upbringing in the faith emphasized the importance of forgiving transgressions. However, much of this forgiveness involved understanding that Christ possesses the supernatural power to forgive our sins. Yet it's a different ball game regarding our conflict to forgive ourselves. It is easier for me to believe in a God who forgives out of love, but it remains much harder for me to forgive on a personal level.

What I've come to learn and practice daily is that when it comes to self-forgiveness, I must reflect on the structure or dynamic of my life at the time my unhealthy choices took the best of me. I'm not coming up with justifications for the choices we might regret. Instead, I'm offering the idea of giving yourself some grace. You were doing what you needed at that moment in your life. And although you may still struggle daily with forgiveness, understand that this process will not be wasted, as it also helps to shape your character.

If I hadn't made mistakes I was ashamed of, I wouldn't have learned how to better myself with introspection and forgiveness. And when you blend the concept of grace and the practice of forgiveness, you begin to feel lighter and more at ease. Which, in turn, teaches you lessons. And being a student in your own life is much more rewarding than cowering behind the fear of not learning.

Before my diagnosis, I kept my wounding hidden. I didn't want others to judge me. I allowed the wounds to edge their way toward scarring because I wasn't working on mending them. I didn't look at these ugly things because they made me feel unattractive. And the more I ignored the pestering thoughts of shame, the more they showed up when I was quiet. My yoga mat would act as an oversized absorbent paper towel where tears could be held and secrets could be hidden. So, when I discovered that I could practice self-forgiveness, I began with trepidation. As I navigated these uncharted waters, I realized I had to actively adjust my internal language. I realized that I was in control of reshaping my thought life as it related to things that brought me shame. And as with most things, practice makes perfect, but in this case, practice made power.

My body felt my movement toward celebrating myself amidst the ugly. It recognized that I was trying to clear dusty and moldy memory vessels of shame, and it was helping to pave the way by restoring one cell of emotion at a time. This is still a significant work in progress for me. But I feel my body, on a deep and cellular level, bowing to me, with walls crumbling all around.

As it is relayed in the book of Mathew, Peter approached Jesus and asked, "Lord, how many times shall I forgive my brother or sister who sins against me? Up to seven times?" Jesus replied, "I tell you, not seven times, but seventy-seven times" (Matthew 18:21-22). I believe Jesus also understood the importance of both external and internal forgiveness for our well-being. Through the exchange between Jesus and Peter, the command for forgiveness is endless. May we be faithful forgivers to ourselves and others, keeping our health as pristine as possible.

December 2022: Joyless Blood

It's December 5th, Charlie and Violet turn eight, and I can leave my 21-day hospital stay. The nurses helped pack my bags and insisted I ride the wheelchair down. I'm annoyed, but it's hospital policy. I'm so over the wheelchair thing. It's such a tease. If it had a personality, it would be like the high school bully who never said anything out loud but instead gave looks and smirks that were ten times worse.

My wheelchair whispered, *Look at you thinking you've got this cancer thing beat. You are leaving the hospital, but not with the confidence you had when you walked in. They won't let you go unless you are with me.*

Therefore, I refuse to put the foot supports up. I dangle my feet to have some thimble of power and hope the nurse doesn't see my subtle defiance.

It's dark out, and I sit in the wheelchair just outside the hospital with my nurse keeping me steady behind. We scan the cars, pulling up until I see my cousin's white minivan. The air is musty and crisp all at the same time. It's busy, with cars, people, and everyone not wanting to be where they are. It's late, and drivers and patients are tired. I keep breathing as much as I can. The thick and dirty air is better than having no air, I have had for the past 21 days. I sink into the passenger seat. My cousin puts her hand on my knee, and I lean forward and weep. I'm used to this by now. I promised myself from the beginning that I would feel as deeply as I could, especially when it came to the widest and deepest of trenches.

My cousin dropped me off at the apartment Kyle and I rented during our separation. My immune system is too fragile to see the kids just yet. I still have to wait a week before I can visit the house. The apartment smells like I remember it. My personal touches are still there to make it feel like it's somewhat of an escape home. I want this first night home to feel as normal as possible. So I ordered a Caprese salad and Grandma's Personal Pie from a local restaurant. I found a Netflix movie, and I'm willing to escape into the simplest joys of life I could think of. I can barely keep my eyes open during the Hallmark-like movie.

The food tastes like I'm eating a mouthful of pennies. I gag, I throw up, and I try again. The nursing staff told me that my taste sensations would return in about six weeks, and I brushed it off, thinking that maybe I would be an anomaly. I wasn't.

Food was my enemy. It taunted me with former tastes until I tasted it. Metallic and sharp shudders radiated through my mouth, and the only way out was to spit my first bite into the garbage. Strawberry Ensures were my go-to, as was Grape Nuts cereal. Weirdly, Grape Nuts cereal was the only food outside my Ensure that I could stomach. I spoke with a bone marrow patient in the hospital who could only eat canned baked beans after her transplant. I'm glad my craving didn't replicate the likes of what cavemen were inclined to eat. My Grape Nuts cereal made me feel a bit more sophisticated.

After a week of my apartment isolation, bad Netflix shows, hour-long trips north for blood checks, and forcing myself to use the

221

bathroom, I am finally given the "okay" to go home and see my kids. But it's a tease. I can't hug, touch, snuggle, or hold them. It was easier not to be with them than to be with them and not be able to experience the "all" of them. These moments are the subtleties of blood cancer recovery that make this disease so emotionally penetrable. I sit on the couch in my living room, wearing double masks, and watch my kids. The couch is arranged around the Christmas tree. It's the tree I decorated with them on November 13th. The day before, I was admitted for my transplant.

That same day, Violet and I pumped out six dozen Christmas cookies, which I tucked away in the freezer. I was determined to make sure that when I came home from the hospital, all the things that made Christmas special would still be there.

What I didn't realize was that I couldn't fully be there. I couldn't keep my eyes open for more than 45 minutes. I retreated to my bedroom hourly to get enough rest to make it through another hour. Kyle was gracious and understood my inability to complete the simplest tasks. I spend the days with my kids, but return to the apartment around 5 pm to get some sleep.

It's a regular night of quiet, lousy TV, strawberry Ensure, and lemonade Crystal Light, as I still couldn't stomach water. My shoulder hurts, and I chalk it up to stress and muscle tension. But it gets worse quickly. My arm starts to swell, and the pain is pulsing up and down my arm. A fever begins, and I know that something is wrong. My wrist started to expand, and I had to cut off two of the bracelets Stella had made for me for my birthday and Mother's Day. And it's in that moment of frantically releasing the tension of the bracelets that I have the intuitive awareness that I am working against a blood clot.

My dad is in town as he's the grandparent on-call this week. I make the phone call, and he's at the apartment in five minutes. He breaks his 10-mile speed limit rule and fast-tracks me an hour north to the hospital where my transplant took place. He's quiet, and I'm crying. Partly out of physical pain, but mostly out of pain and anger.

He lets me yell, curse, and punch the dashboard. "What the hell?! Why are all these shitty things happening to me?!"

We arrive. He drops me off at the ER door while cars behind us honk with irritation that we are holding up traffic for 30 seconds. Almost in unison and in the same intonation, we tell the stranger behind us to shut up. It's disturbingly similar, and I know we both get a kick out of this. A silent connection that reminds the two of us that we are made from the same hot-blooded Italian thread.

The ER is bustling. Standing room only. I push myself through the crowd, piss people off, and make my way to the front of the line. I hold the green Bone Marrow Transplant card, which will forever be in my wallet, and I request a room with isolation through the plexiglass shield, likely installed during the COVID days. The receptionist has obnoxious, yellow, and gold-tipped nails that are far too long for her fingers. I'm judging her, and I don't even know her. She asks me to wait for my name, but I refuse to.

My dad stands a few feet away, allowing me to handle the situation. I'm glad he's allowing me to handle this situation on my own. I glare at the receptionist and wonder how she might feel if she had to

223

wear a cancer beanie on a cold December night. I tuck myself away from the crowd as far as possible and wait for my name to be called.

My foot is twitching, and my anger is boiling. I'm licking my lips, gritting my teeth, and taking shallow breaths beneath my double masks. I have zero immunity and am immersed in a cluster- fuck of hazardous germs. I make a side glance at my dad. His arms are crossed, and he stands strong but helpless. He is also aware of the situation.

And through it all, I am incredibly grateful that he allows me to take the reins in this situation. I glare at the receptionist until I can't stand it any longer. I march with confidence to that stupid plexiglass shield, piss more people off and say, "If you don't get me in there, you are compromising the life of someone who hopes to continue this life."

Soon after, I'm admitted into an isolated room where my dad feels free to cry, and I feel free to ask for the drugs I know will alleviate my pain. The nurses listen to me. They are too busy not to, and they know that I'm a fragile case. I'm not there for stitches or to assist a croup-coughing toddler. They know I don't have the schooling, but they know that I have a failed immune system, which knows what synthetic concoction of a drug can keep my system at ease for now. I ask, they deliver, and I get through the next seven hours until a room is available.

It's 3 am. I tell my dad to go home. He doesn't want to, and I get that. I'm not a 44-year-old strong bald woman to him. I'm a six-year-old with pin-straight braids who always followed the rules. Eventually, he leaves, and my heart aches for him as I envision leaving one of my children in this situation.

I spent five "bonus" days in the hospital post-transplant due to the blood clot I suspected. My doctor confidently assured me that this was my "one thing." All bone marrow transplant patients encounter one major hiccup after the procedure. She says it with assurance, and I trust her. I've always trusted her. And it's curious to me because she's just human. I'm unsure whether it's due to my naivety or because I trust her expertise. Either way, I'll take the hiccup of a blood clot in my jugular vein that is still being monitored ten months post-diagnosis.

I know that blood is life and that my blood has been stripped of life for far too long. It's old blood, bad blood, tainted blood, and has for far too long been joyless blood. I am in the middle of a rebirth. It makes sense that the old blood is jealous of the new blood and will do its best to stop the process of new life regenerating.

I return to the apartment, representing everything that has fallen apart. A broken marriage, a place to recover from a life-saving procedure, and solace from a world I so desperately want to be a part of. My visiting nurse makes two weekly house calls and changes my port dressings. I look forward to these visits. Her careful cleaning, precision, and care in redressing the bandages feel so good —a feeling akin to crawling into freshly made bed sheets after a long day. I'm hooked up to an IV, which contains a constant Magnesium drip. I don't care much about this inconvenience. It's a minimal annoyance in the scheme of all I've been through.

It's Christmas morning. I set my alarm for 5 am so that I can arrive at the house to sit quietly for an hour before little feet pound the floor. I plan this hour because it's one of the best hours of the year. When I was young, I made it a tradition to read The Velveteen

225

Rabbit to pass the time while I waited for my parents to say it was okay to come to the tree. That's me, an old soul who can't skip out on tradition.

I'm proud of myself this Christmas. And it's not just because I'm here. I knew I would be here. I had the wherewithal to order, wrap, and hide the gifts in early November with the self-awareness that all would be set when I arrived home. Christmas was always meaningful in my home growing up. It may sound simplistic to say this day always felt magical, but it did. The smells, the paper, and gifts that disappointed you all played a role in a day that felt like nothing could go wrong. The day after that was always a subtle letdown. Every kid knows this, anticipates, and gets through that day as best they can. I still feel this way, even as an adult.

I take in every smile, laugh, and grudge from tired teens as they open their gifts. I'm exhausted, and I've only been up an hour. I adjust my beanie and double masks and sit in the far corner of the couch so I'm not too close to them. All I can think about is getting back into bed. And that's Christmas Day for me. Twenty minutes awake and an hour asleep. It's a song and dance of trying to blend into the prior experience while tenderly caring for my new immune system, which is working on overdrive. In many ways, I feel more dead than alive, and that makes me mad. There is absolutely nothing I can do to change this lifeless feeling into something more productive.

The only thing my Charlie was hoping for from Santa was a $12 styrofoam airplane. I was so proud of him for wanting such a simple toy. The kind of toy I grew up with. Similar to a Jack-in-the-Box or

Mr. Potato Head. A handheld toy that he could manipulate and trust not to break, as there weren't any electronic components involved.

Later in the afternoon, I feel energized enough to go to the beach with Kyle, the dog, and the kids. Charlie clutches his airplane the entire ride as he anticipates trying it out on the vastness of the beach. We arrive, and he runs ahead, launching the plane. It nosedives immediately. He's not frustrated, and he keeps trying. And eventually, he gets it. He begins to manipulate how he holds it to make it twist and turn. I admire his little boy spirit and know how much I will miss it someday.

And that's when it happens.

He overthrows and misjudges his proximity to the water. It seemed as if the plane was moving in slow motion, nose first into the waves. He watches, he's paralyzed, and then he screams. There it is. A $12, red, styrofoam airplane ordered from Amazon just suspended out there at the will of the ocean's decision.

He runs to the water and stops knee-deep. He's crying, and his eyes won't move from the red floating object. He cannot do anything but hope that it may move toward him. And I ache with him because it's kind of how I feel. I'm out there suspended and at the mercy of the medicine, the donor cells, and my doctors, all in hopes that I will reach shore safely.

I sit beside Charlie and explain that Santa has a backup plan in place for such incidents. It's called Amazon. We order the red airplane as he watches his original float away. He's clever enough to understand now that Santa isn't real, and I'm all the wiser knowing that backup plans are often better in disguise.

Truth 31: Grieve Hard

June 26, 2024

The more we dictate to ourselves what we should do and how we should process loss, the more we suffocate the cellular part of ourselves that is imperative to our emotional growth.

Thousands of books have been written about grief, the stages of grief, and any and everything related to helping ourselves and others. But nothing written in a text or said by a trained therapist is going to fill the void of losing someone in your life that you love. Our body screams inside; our blood feels like fire when the loss occurs. Losing someone you love is like losing a piece of yourself, and the orchestra of life will miss a beautiful note from that point on.

I come from a large Italian family on my dad's side. Salted meats, pastiche, anisettes, and everyone talking over one another can pretty much summarize any family gathering. Aunts and Uncles feel like moms and dads. Cousins feel like sisters and brothers. If someone is affected, it affects all of us, and within minutes, we get the phone calls, read the texts, and are all on the same page. This is family. And I am forever grateful to my nosy, food-loving, and faith-living family.

I hadn't planned on including this truth in my notes while preparing for this book. I didn't include it because I haven't had to practice grieving hard until now. My family is shaken; we are all crying in some form today as my beautiful Aunt Donna is being put on hospice care today as a result of a sudden stroke six days ago.

And just like that, the curve ball of life, the plot twist that takes your breath away. I call my sister and cousin and navigate how awful this is. And I'm angry. I'm so angry that the people I love the most are hurting the hardest. This is my first taste of loss, and I don't know what my body is doing. Memories swirl, crying follows, confusion, and then release. And I understand that my body, my cells, are all readjusting to unexpected emotional chaos I'm trying to figure out. But that's the thing: I don't have to figure it out. I have to give my body the space to learn grief in the ways that it needs. I don't hold it together in front of my kids or tell people I'm fine. No rules and barricades are set up within the walls of my heart on how much I'm allowed to grieve.

When we honor our process of grief, we are celebrating the person we lost. This person would not want to see you escaping to unhealthy choices to numb the endless ache of loss. This person, if they could, would like to hold you as you cried until your throat was raw. The more we dictate to ourselves what we should do and how we should process loss, the more we suffocate the cellular part of ourselves that is imperative to our emotional growth. Our bodies will use all experiences, happy and sad, to our benefit. We think we have to control our reactions to things, and there is a place for that. But I believe that when it comes to losing someone you love, you are doing your health a disservice if you don't feel the pain in the way that your body requires.

I will miss my Aunt Donna's sweet smile, soft hugs, and the love I felt when I was around her. And that was who she was. She was love. And I don't think I can process much more right now because my hands are too shaky to type. So, I will end this truth short because I'm learning to handle only what I can.

To grieve hard means to feel everything. It means to cry, yell, or be still. There is no rule book for how you should be. You honor this person when you honor yourself in this way. They applaud your intuitiveness from the heavens through daily and subtle reminders of their presence. You will see.

Truth 32: Four Friends

You only need four friends; each has a different place and purpose.

I was probably around 6 or 7 when the world unabashedly informed me that friendships aren't as honest as you would hope. I was at the age of innocence and play. My second-grade class didn't yet hold stock in the prom king and queen status. Those constructs come along around the fifth grade. We were just kids running around like bees from a hive on a hot, blacktop elementary school playground. My memory is vivid and has affected me deeply.

I'm on the playground with one of my friends, though I cannot remember who or the specifics. But I remember her reaching into her pocket and pulling out two shiny, cheap necklaces. They were friendship necklaces, and I had never seen anything like them. Each cheap silver chain held half of a heart that, when locked together, created a whole heart with the words inscribed "best friends." One side was pink, and the other side was purple. I quickly connected the dots and understood that the two who shared these necklaces were "bosom buddies," similar to Anne and Diana in the classic series written by L.M. Montgomery. And I felt light inside, beyond excited to share this sacred connection with my new best friend. And that was the first time I was introduced to the concept of a "best" friend. I had no idea what it meant other than that this friend would pick ME to be her friend, chosen above others.

And then it happened. I felt gut pain when I watched her approach another classmate and excitedly hand her half of the necklace. They took turns clasping the necklaces around each other. I stood there defeated, rejected, and overwhelmingly confused. I wasn't angry or jealous; I was just sad. Since then, I haven't believed in best friends because, at some point, your heart will likely be broken, and you won't be able to find the purple half of your pink.

We live in a world where our social connections occur while scrolling through a screen in a doctor's office waiting room. We comment on funny Instagram reels sent by friends while sitting on the couch at 8 pm. Mini, meaningless, surface-based connections all day long. And even though we might have 976 friends on our Facebook page and our Instagram account has 800 followers, there isn't anything of emotional depth regarding these numbers, as much as these tools make it feel like we are connecting. Instead, we are disintegrating our time abilities to practice being human with another human. Our emotional reactions are shared through prayer hands, sad faces, and heart emojis. It pains me that my children are growing up in a world where passing notes to one another in class and knocking on doors to play seem so outdated.

As I navigate my adult life, I am daily reminded that one of my most precious resources is my time. And how I choose to spend that time is entirely up to me. We have 24 hours a day to work, sleep, make social connections, and do a million other things. And what a shame it would be if I were actively connecting with many people on a superficial level rather than an emotionally invested level. I don't have time to waste on people who won't challenge me and hold me accountable to the standards I set for myself. It might sound selfish, but if you want to stay healthy for yourself, be sure to stay selfish for yourself. With that said, I have developed the Four Friends recipe. It's simple. You only need four friends; each has a different place and purpose. Since my sickness, I have applied my clever philosophy, which has resulted in protecting my energy and increasing my trust in others.

Everyone needs a Foundational Friend. This is the friend that you met in first grade. You went on overnight Boy Scout or Girl Scout camping trips. You playfully teased each other, were experts at pretend play, and asked parents for sleepovers as often as possible. Your friendship continues through middle school, and though it might have been rocky, you figure it out. High school arrives, and you attend proms together. You sneak out to your first party with this friend. This friend is the secret keeper of your limited world of juvenile drama. This friend will always be your friend. You will meet at a high school reunion years later and feel as though the aging process wasn't possible, as yesterday you were wrinkle-free and nothing ached. This friend isn't a best friend. This friend was placed in your life to help you learn who you are and what you want to become as you look to the future.

The next friend you need is a realist friend. This is the one who keeps you grounded. You can come to this friend with relationship problems, grandiose ideas of starting a business, or tears of self-doubt and depression. This friend is solid. They care about you, but more importantly, they know they have a job. They know that humans need humans. And as much as you need your realist friend, they also need you. You need this person in your life because they won't lie to you; instead, they offer the hard truth of what you need to hear, rather than what you want to hear. They play the vital role of challenging your way of thinking. They like to ruffle your feathers a bit to get you thinking. This is not done out of malice but instead out of love. They are part of your chosen protection plan. Whether or not you take their advice, they are there to challenge the go-to ways of thinking that your formative years might have missed.

I remember walking into my first therapy appointment in college. I was scared to death. I had no idea what was expected of me or how everything would unfold. But I was put at ease when the therapist immediately said, "You can talk, and I will listen. And if you don't want to talk, that's okay too, but I will be here if you change your mind." So I did that. I sat there for a while, staring at my foot, which was encased in a brown sandal, and twitching anxiously with my legs crossed. Every subtle indicator of body language suggested that I didn't want to be there. But as the minutes passed and he did as promised, I felt my body soften and slowly begin to trust this stranger. And this was the first time I learned what it meant to hold someone's space because that's exactly what he was doing for me.

Everyone needs a space-holder friend. This friend is important because they carry the sacred calling of holding your energy with their presence. They appear detached from their problems, which humans often struggle with. This friend is hard to find, but when you do find them, you will know. They can feel your energy without many words and guide you by doing almost nothing. Because through their nothing, there is everything. Being in their presence makes you feel safe and allows the answers to come to you. You sit with this person in a nest of energy where you feel protected and trust a friend willing to be there for you. I look forward to meeting this friend someday.

And lastly, everyone needs a seasonal friend. Scripture states, "There is a time for everything and a season for every activity under the heavens" (Ecclesiastes 3:1). I think we can apply this wisdom to our friendships. It makes sense that as we transition through the many seasons of our lives, the right people will come alongside and support us in our child-rearing and then our empty-nester days. Our life is riddled with changes at so many different intersections. Moving to a new place, changing jobs, starting a new relationship, and letting go of other ones. People cross our paths daily, and our intuition and vibrations attract those who are meant to walk beside us for a time before moving on to walk beside another.

I've found through my experience that seasonal friends work their magic in your life for about 5-7 years. And when this friendship ends, it's not abrupt or damaging. It's a knowing and a natural agreement without words that you have both fulfilled the contract of friendship your lives needed during that season. This friend can feel like a best friend, but they are not. They are not your best friend because others who come after them will also feel like best friends. This is why I do not believe in the idea of a best friend. And maybe I'm wrong on this one, given my inability to trust anyone. Either way, I'm not down for wearing one half of a necklace just in case the other person loses their half.

Keep your circle small. And as someone once said, "It's better to have four quarters than 100 pennies."

Truth 33: It's Your Story

Each of us is like a walking library; we have books with chapters we like to revisit, and we knowingly leave others on their dusty shelves.

One of my favorite things to do in the summer is watching people walk the boardwalk. Benches align the sandy boards, most engraved with the name of a loved one no longer here. I find a bench, sink in, and watch the parade of people, families, and kids dodging in and out of the crowd, ice cream cones in hand like a speeding car down the parkway.

Most of these people are from out of town and vacationing with their families at the peak of the summer. I love seeing the dynamic of older and younger eyes taking in our small but fun boardwalk. Kids who wear water shoes with white zinc smeared beneath their eyes are likely at the beach for the first time, and I smile inside. I smile because the ocean has a distinct energy that brings people together with one common theme in mind. The theme is that we are all unknowingly more present with ourselves and each other from the moment we step onto the well-worn boards.

And while I soak up this summer scene, I wonder about the stories these people carry. The hard stories, the love stories, the sad stories, and the joy stories. Each of us is like a walking library; we have books with chapters we like to revisit, and we knowingly leave others on their dusty shelves.

The problem is that often, we are the only ones who know about these stories. We don't share our stories for a variety of reasons. The stories that carry shame make us cower as we want to protect our appearance. The stories embedded with guilt cannot be shared out of fear of judgment. If shared, the stories that carry fear might bring disappointment from the ones closest to us. But these are the stories worth sharing that others need to hear. And just as I've shared about vulnerability, the same truth applies here.

The more we peel back the layers to our raw and authentic selves, the more space we allow others to do the same. We hide our stories behind vacation posts on Facebook, which no one cares about anyway. Some of us hide our stories on the same barstool in town and, maybe, occasionally, share a few sentences with the bartender. Others hide their stories by appearing to be the best at something. The key word is "appearing," as it's often the moms who go over the top with perfectly themed birthday parties or the men with the biggest boats who are the ones with the most painful stories carrying the most dust.

One of the biggest lessons cancer has taught me is that people need people. During my 49-day isolation at Jersey Shore Medical Center, followed by 21-day isolation at Hackensack Medical Center, I felt my soul self disintegrating without daily face-to-face, meaningful connections with other humans. Nurses and doctors understood the loneliness part of this disease and tried to connect with me through mini conversations unrelated to blood counts. I was grateful for that. But they were busy, and I could read their body language as they needed to be elsewhere. They didn't want to diminish my presence as just a patient but as a human stripped away from her foundation. Her children.

People ask me what was most challenging about this disease, and I will always say loneliness. This is saying a lot, as bone marrow biopsies are painful. I wish on no one.

So, if loneliness was the most challenging part of my journey, what is the healing agent that brings a cure? It's people, it's connection, it's being vulnerable, it's creating space for two people to listen to each other's stories and discover ways that support their growth. I live with intention now and try to be as transparent as possible. There is no reason not to be. Choosing to lock the door to your ever-expanding library produces nothing. But reading a few pages here and there will help others, and yourself learn lessons that could never be discovered.

We are called to share our stories. It's time to stop feeling ashamed and expecting judgment where there might not be any. We are human, fallen, and all a mess; nobody knows what they're doing. We move through the motions of life, hoping we stay healthy and keep our jobs, and we often know that the next shoe will drop soon. But healing comes with sharing, and doors you didn't even know were available begin to open themselves.

Your story is powerful. Own it. Stand firm in knowing that what you have to share is important, and as one close friend told me, "Sarah, what you write will be liked by at least one person." And that's all you need—one person. The energy created by two people sharing two different stories can bring forth a novel of life lessons we couldn't learn on our own.

You will know when to share part or all of your story. Life will present opportunities for you to read the entire chapter or just a few pages to another trusted person. Allow the universe to guide you and trust the process. We go through hard times so that we can be an encouragement to others on their journey. Don't be selfish with your hard. Make it your friend. The more you embrace it, the harder it is for it to hold you completely. Be brave with your storytelling. It's yours to share and others to learn from.

Truth 34: Discipline Delivers

Discipline is a learned practice that, when applied toward your biggest dream, can unlock the potential for greatness.

The things that produce the greatest results are the things that require the most attention, also known as discipline. There will never be an athlete participating at the national level who does not live with discipline in their training, diet, mindset, and sleep. There will never be a musician on a world-renowned stage who does not practice and refine his instrument daily. And there will not be an author who produces a book if she puts off her time with her laptop. Discipline is learned, practiced, and incredibly hard to maintain. Many would say that I'm a very disciplined individual. I agree with them, even though my discipline can sometimes hinder my ability to roll with things. Some might disagree, but the nature/nurture principle applies here. I don't believe we are born disciplined. I think it's something learned and practiced. And if we are introduced to this character trait early, it lends itself to bigger things later.

I was raised on a farm and had many responsibilities. The 16-year-old sophomore, who gave water to her horses at 6:30 am before school, was irritated with this requirement, but in the end, the discipline of simple chores like this helped shape my character. I was a nationally ranked athlete, and with that came extreme discipline related to the type of training and rest I put in on a weekly basis. Although I disliked the sport while participating in it, I am grateful for the discipline it instilled in me. If I were to take the extensive definition of how discipline benefits us and sift it through a colander of understanding, I would say this:

Discipline is a learned practice that, when applied toward your biggest goal, can unlock the potential for greatness.

Without sounding like a cheesy Facebook quote, I plan to relay my ideas about our dreams and goals more sophisticatedly. We are introduced to the idea of our dreams coming true through elementary school assemblies aimed at forming our character, led by motivational skits of twenty-somethings who graduated from college with a theater degree. This idea of "anything is possible if you follow your dreams" was reinforced through teachers, parents, music, well-worn classroom posters on concrete walls, and several other sources. But there came a point in our early adult life when we realized these words of potential felt like just words. But for others, it was real, penetrable, and something we held loosely at first and then tightly to when we started to see the results that discipline exerted toward achieving a goal.

When we honor our human potential and instill gifts, we align with the truth of who we are and what we are meant to do here. The problem is that the world's weight gets in the way of what we see ourselves achieving while admiring others who find their way to the finish line of self-empowerment. We all have essential responsibilities as parents, business owners, and employees. I do not dispute our commitment to these roles. But I do believe that if you feel something substantial, something that might be something, something that you are called to create, it's there that you make space to work on it. And that's where discipline comes in.

My question for you is this. What do you feel gifted in, and what would that look like if you saw yourself in the highest position while utilizing this gift? This is a loaded question, and I feel pressured as I deliver this challenge. However, when we boil this concept down, it is there that we begin to understand the undiscovered power. The world stifles it with all the "to-do" lists and the "shoulds," but it's up to the individual to step into bravery and do something with their unique talents.

The recipe for success is straightforward. It's twenty minutes a day. That's all it is. If you can find space in at least five out of seven days a week to devote 20 minutes, you will be on the path toward your goal. And while putting in the reps toward your dream, you begin to envision a greater purpose of self and feel propelled to do more. You start to see yourself beyond the societal roles expected of you. It becomes part of you; you don't need to explain it to others because you already know how powerful it is. I've learned through hard lessons not to share too much with people. They talk. They are not affirming. And they are doubtful. And you do not need to doubt. You must stay true to who you are called to be and trust the process, not the people around you.

When you give energy to what you love, you provide the Universe with more power to help you achieve a goal that would be harder to achieve through your blueprint of ideas. I think about the greats of music. I imagine most of them began in the basement or garage of their parents' home. They had a vision, a dream, an idea that they might someday be somebody. They didn't know how this would happen; they just kept enjoying their love for a dream coming true while participating in the unfolding script. For a very few, that dream has come true. For others, it does not. Is this discipline talent or a combination of both? I don't know. But there's a treasure and a beauty in the process that, if not explored, one will never experience. What I do know is that the greats are where they are because they cultivated their gifts and then gave these gifts time and attention through disciplined dedication.

I challenge you to get quiet and ask yourself what you envision yourself accomplishing or striving toward that might be one step further toward your full potential. In this thought process, you need to become a little selfish. In this case, selfishness is necessary. You are the most important human in the world. What you feed, your soul will flourish. What you choose to withhold will diminish what you could become. It's important not to focus on the long road to reach a destination; instead, take the next small step. And if you devote just twenty minutes a day, five times a week, you will spend 80 hours a year working toward what you truly value. And nothing concrete may come from your dedication, and that's okay. Because what you have learned along the way is the process of discipline and character development.

Even as I feverishly type these words, thinking this book might be something, I realize it might not. But I'm okay with that. Through this process of discipline, I'm finding a better version of myself. Learning about yourself helps us better relate to the world around us. Understanding how we respond, react, and evaluate is huge for self-growth.

Find your gift, and don't be afraid to dip pieces of your soul into where it could lead. As referenced in the book of Esther, "And who knows but that you have come to your royal position for such a time as this?" (Esther 4:14). You will know your time, you will hear the whispers, and if brave enough, you will begin to explore your potential. And this potential is refined through discipline and vision. Both go hand in hand, and they are thought about daily. Make this call a part of who you were created to be. The world will be a more complete place if you dare to be both intuitive and disciplined in your calling.

Truth 35: Broken is Beautiful

The redeeming part is that, as despairing as the pieces may appear on the floor, rebuilding the art of your life introduces the finer gifts of you...The artist.

In fourth grade, my class took a field trip to the Clark Art Institute in Williamstown, MA. Up until then, I had never given art much thought. Art was a class we took in school, and the result was an attempted replication of Van Gogh's Starry Night. The trip held an unexpected discovery that I wasn't prepared for. I was introduced to Winslow Homer. I looked at his work, his strokes, the movement of the water, the boats, and the people. I don't know what about his work had an impact, and to this day, I still don't know. My parents gave me $10 to spend at the museum gift shop, and I willingly spent all of my money on Winslow Homer postcards. I wanted to remember what I felt when I looked at his work, not what I saw. This reminds us of the simple lesson that we remember how people make us feel, not what they do for us. Winslow Homer made a 10-year-old girl, who knew almost nothing about art, feel things that are still beyond her definition.

I am forever grateful for my 22-year marriage to Kyle for several reasons. There are too many to count. People are put in our lives to teach us lessons; he has been one of my biggest teachers. I will always love Kyle, and he knows that. But we both agreed that the type of love we were trying to cling to had long since vaporized. One of his most prominent influences was introducing art into my life. I vividly remember falling in love with him while he painted my portrait. He was a graduate art student at the University of

Delaware, where he was awarded a studio to work in. I would make the five-hour drive from upstate NY to visit whenever possible. His studio was cluttered, with canvas and tubes of paint of different shapes and colors scattered around. Art studios carry a particular scent that is both welcoming and off-putting at the same time. I'll always think of Kyle when the faint smell of oil paint finds its way to me. Walls were covered in drawings and paintings, some from other artists or those he admired. As a new college graduate of 22 with stars in her eyes, this was so incredibly romantic for me. I was sure to sit very still while wearing a light blue and white embroidered shirt I had purchased for this sitting from Old Navy. I still have that shirt in my closet.

Kyle challenged me to give all different kinds of art a chance. Instead of dismissing pieces of work, I didn't understand, he prompted me to sit with the painting or sculpture, study it, and then notice how it made me feel. Art, like writing, tells a story, and it's through the strokes that the artist's power is transferred to you. However, you must be open to receiving. And that's exactly what happened with Mr. Homer's "Breezing Up (A Fair Wind)," created in 1873.

A few years ago, I came across a type of art called Kintsugi. It's a Japanese art form that symbolizes heartache, grief, and difficult times, beautifully redeeming them. Similar to a phoenix rising from the ashes. As scripture states, "I will turn their mourning into gladness; I will give them comfort and joy instead of sorrow" (Jeremiah 31:13). If we imagine ourselves as a beautiful piece of pottery, no blemishes, smooth as glass, and untainted, it's due time before this pottery creates a crack or worse shatters into pieces.

246

Kintsugi art involves repairing a vessel, such as a pot or a vase, or even jewelry, by mending the pieces together with gold, silver, or platinum, and creating a piece of art that is far more valuable than when it was first created. The lesson here is that when we were born as an untainted soul, it was predestined for us that the heaviness of the world would break us. This is part of the journey. Unfortunately, most of us don't feel brave enough to share our brokenness. Shame and guilt play a significant role here, but bravery ultimately prevails over both. Hiding behind our sadness only produces more tears, and surrendering to disappointment in ourselves only pushes us deeper into caves of unworthiness.

When we begin to own, share, and embrace our mistakes, it is here that we are made more beautiful. Self-forgiveness is practiced, making the process a double bonus. Instead of seeing the hard things as stagnant and defining, challenge yourself to see them as blessings in disguise.

Cancer was hard. However, my hard work is different from yours. Collectively, this hard is all the same. It can't be measured with the invisible ruler of life that we think we need to apply. Let's begin to translate the hard into the beautiful. Let's experiment with wearing a lens that presents a human who makes mistakes and turns that into a stronger and wiser human for that moment or choice made. Bottom line...you are going to screw up, and hard times are going to come. Accept it. Trying to navigate this life without hiccups along the way is far-fetched and impossible. It is much easier to embrace the fact that I don't have all the answers and that I will continue to screw up. Knowingly at times and unknowingly at other times. The redeeming part is that, as despairing as the pieces may appear on the floor, the process of rebuilding the art of your life introduces the finer gifts of you...The artist.

You know what it is that you are ashamed of. You know what you wish you could redo. You may be in unrest and battling something that seems too big to tackle. Trust me when I say this. The tighter you embrace this hard thing or mistake, the more beautiful you become. And the beauty results from repairing these things with lessons of gold throughout the process. Gold is a gift, and it's given on special occasions. You are a special occasion. Start accepting the repair with the finest of metals. The result is a more valuable you. And when you begin to share your repair process with others, you open the doors for the other person to discover the artist within them.

Be a little different. Different is good. Share your ugly, share your shame, share your mistakes. God has you. The Universe has you. It's waiting for you to feel all sparkly and pretty, as gold will run through your veins.

Truth 36: Quit Judging

When we set aside our tendency to judge others, we nurture the castle of character we are building within ourselves.

The older I get, the more curious I become about my upbringing in my born-again Christian faith. As a child, I didn't know what a formal church looked like. I drove by them as my mom brought me to piano lessons and cross-country races, but I had never seen the inner workings. I had never been in a Church because my family was part of what we called The Home Fellowship. Each Sunday was spent in a different home. Our family hosted it on the third Sunday of each month. Our home served as the church, and attendees would start rolling in a little before 10 am. The service involved music, sharing, and reading aloud passages from the bible that had touched individuals in some personal way the week preceding. The congregation of people I faithfully attended each Sunday loved one another. It felt like a family, and I was okay with it because I didn't know any other way to live my faith.

Despite the blurred lines of my religious upbringing, I continue to reflect upon this type of worship. I am grateful for being introduced to a deeper understanding of Christ on a personal level. The Home Fellowship will forever be a formative part of my character, even if it means repeatedly learning about Noah's Ark in Sunday school.

When writing this book, I decided not to hold anything against my parents or extended family who were part of the Fellowship. It was our church; it was what we knew, and I admire my parents for their faithful dedication. However, with any faith, there are aspects that we need to examine to decide for ourselves if this is what we are meant to hold onto. There's a lot I can write about and reflect on, along with questions, when I sift through the memories of my church upbringing. However, one theme that seems to thread itself throughout the words of scripture is the ugly word called judgment.

As a child, I viewed Jesus, God, and the Holy Spirit, also known as the Trinity, as one person. But I feared this dynamic trio so much that I didn't feel love. I felt watched, pinned in a corner if I made a bad choice, and fearful. The numerous times I re-dedicated my life to Christ during my childhood are almost comical. I felt like I was never good enough, never blameless, always on the edge of "What if I die today and go to hell because I didn't confess that I lied to my parents earlier that day?" It was a conflict in my 9-year-old brain because, at home fellowship, we sang songs about forgiveness, love, and washing away our sins, but the greater emphasis always seemed to be saving lost souls, and we being one of them.

And it was there that I was introduced to judgment. I didn't know it then, but upon reflection, we were a very judgmental group of people. Judgment on those in the congregation who had been divorced. Judgment on those who chose a gay or lesbian lifestyle. Judgment to those who had extramarital affairs and came clean about them. Judgment toward those who were flooded with tattoos and nose rings. Judgment toward someone who made the difficult decision to abort a child. The list goes on and on and on. Please note that I will not impose my opinions on these topics. Instead, I will share what my child self saw, felt, and what it led to, causing me to feel conflicted about. If we were singing about a God of love, why were we being so hard on the people who most needed love?

We all struggle with our immediate reaction to judge other people. We are constantly comparing, gossiping, and more worried about someone else's drama than being reflective. Instead, we should be working on our own drama! That's funny about becoming more involved in other people's worlds. It's a clever way to ignore and avoid our issues. Isn't talking about someone else's disparity or choices more fun than sharing our own? It is. And the life principle of "what you feed grows" applies well here. The more you find yourself judging, the deeper it becomes embedded in your cellular self. We all have that one friend who gets excited when they have something juicy to talk about. I listen, try not to give away too much energy, and quickly rein myself back if I find myself going down that road. I've learned over time that as soon as I fall into old patterns of faith-based judgment, I ask myself to view this person or this situation for who they are, rather than what it is. It's simple.

People are human, and things happen. People make choices, and things happen. The more imperfect or broken people appear, the more curious I am about them. It's those people that I gravitate to, and I believe Christ would gravitate to them as well. He didn't move His way through scripture, judging and condemning. He walked with open arms to all who would choose to return the embrace. He extended grace, and He forgave quickly. He did not enter a crowd with eyes scanning for sinners and mocking unbelievers. Instead, He wanted to become friends with the lost and wounded. Judgment wouldn't produce healing with someone He was trying to befriend. That would go nowhere.

Each day, you are granted a certain amount of energy. This energy, this life force, is gifted to you to help you decide how to use it. As much as we would like to create more time in a day, a month, or a

251

year, we can't. Time is the one constant that we cannot change or alter. Therefore, the time we spend during our days should be aimed at producing healthy thoughts and promising outcomes. Judging others is wasted energy. There is nothing that comes from it. When we judge, we prove to ourselves that we have weaknesses we refuse to acknowledge. The only reason to judge another human is in a gymnastics-type competition or an area of study where points are applied. Judging humans based on how "we" think they should live their lives is entirely backward. The energy we expend when making speculations and, at times, false accusations about others detracts from our life process. But we do this to feel powerful. This is a false power. We create a sense of importance to ourselves and then appear important to others. Stop judging. If you judge anything in this world, it should be yourself!

Begin to look at other humans as people just trying to live without people like you involved. The challenge is simple but challenging at the same time. Strive to walk as Christ walked. Walk in love and walk without judgment. The less you judge, the more you will welcome. People don't want to be fixed. They want to be seen. They want you to look at them and validate their messiness and their beauty at the same time. And they will reveal this to you when you reveal it to them. Christ walked among the people. This is what made him who he was. He was one of us. Humans do not feel safe among strangers. They feel secure in those they trust. Be the human who consistently creates space for another human without allowing judgment to sneak in.

The Bible uses its melody of text to share its point of view on judgment in a pretty powerful way:

"Do not judge, or you too will be judged. In the same way you judge others, you will be judged, and the measure you use will be measured by you. Why do you look at the speck of sawdust in your brother's eye and pay no attention to the plank in your own eye? How can you tell your brother, 'Let me take the speck out of your eye,' when there is a plank in your own eye all the time? You hypocrite, first take the plank out of your own eye, and then you will see clearly to remove the plank in your brother's eye." (Matthew 7:1-5)

When we set aside our tendency to judge others, we nurture the castle of character we are building within ourselves. That character is yours to create, and with anything, the more you practice releasing the habits of judgment, the more proficient you become with this practice. Similar to my uncanny recollection of the details of Noah's Ark. It was practiced—a lot.

January 2023: Toxic Confetti

It's January 1st, but that date means nothing to me. Instead, the number 41 means everything. I am 41 days post-transplant and almost halfway to reaching the 100-day goal. Every bone marrow patient will recall with trepidation how cautiously we move through these first 100 days. Doctors constantly remind us that we are adult bodies with newborn blood, untainted, and no immunizations. We are the most fragile porcelain dolls, where one hairline fracture or crack could crumble into a thousand pieces.

Day 100 isn't the magical day when I can live and fully put all this behind me. It's just a tiny milestone of assurance that things are still moving forward. I am well aware that I still have 23 months of recovery before this hell is all just a part of the pages of this book. November 21, 2024, is the rainbow's end, and I'll get there. I don't want to celebrate that day. I don't want to go to some tropical island. I don't want to do anything that marks me as an achiever. I want to visit Brennan 6, the Oncology floor at Jersey Shore Medical Center, and hug my nurses. I then want to drive to Hackensack Meridian Hospital alone and hug those nurses. That's all I need. Human connection is everything. Medicine plays a major role in all of this, but medicine doesn't work if the ones administering it don't believe in the process. How many nursing scrubs have I left tears on? So many.

Kyle is in between semesters during January, which works out well. He doesn't complain about driving up north twice a week for my blood tests. I'm not allowed to drive yet because my platelet count is too low, and the risk of bleeding out in a car crash is a harsh reality.

Besides, I'm tired. And it's not just a tired feeling on Sunday afternoon. It's a whole body, exhausted, with every cell screaming to press on. These rides are always quiet, as there isn't much for us to talk about. We are okay with the silence; he knows I would make these drives for him. "Until death do us part" takes on a new meaning for me. He will always be my person until death "does" part us. I never understood divorced couples who treat each other like strangers and slander one another any chance they can get. Because when you peel back the layers of angst and resentment, there are still those early-on remembrances of twenty-something love. So naive, so trusting, and so full of hope. I think it's important to honor the ending of a marriage and simultaneously reflect on the sweetness of its beginning.

Kyle and I joked that we had fallen in love through the Harry Potter series. He would read to me, and I would listen. My head was in his lap while he read with the perfect intonation for each character. I spent hours sitting as a life model for him in his University of Delaware Graduate School art studio. I was 22 years old and dating an artist. My little girl brain thought this was the most romantic thing ever. I loved Kyle, but as a best friend, someone who's always by your side kind of way. That's probably the most difficult sentence for me to write in this book. I still don't know what real love feels like, but I'm learning. And Leukemia is teaching me. Loving the ugly, shameful, and regretful parts of who I am is bringing me into my body for me to understand that I am worthy and will find this real love someday. For now, I *am* love.

I move through January slowly and steadily. Each day starts, and I want it to be over. I go to bed early and sleep in late. I schedule these days in a similar way to my hospital days. It's hour by hour and difficult, as my physical strength is limited. The things my head was telling me I could do ended up disappointing me. My goal was to walk for 30 minutes a day. As a former marathon runner, avid gym-goer, and yoga teacher, I believe these walks would be a highlight of my day. But they are not. I hate them. I hate them because they remind me that I am recovering from a bone marrow transplant. I'm so weak, a shell, and walking to the next mailbox I see is what I focus on.

I bundle up and put on a beanie and two winter hats. I walk slowly, too slowly, and this makes me so angry. Others walk their dogs briskly and smile and nod when they see me. My internal critic wants to scream, "You have no idea how good you have it. Here you are, walking your dog, feeling good, smiling, and checking your phone simultaneously!" Maybe you're headed to a job you hate after walking your dog, but you're still going there.

You don't have to receive any blood transfusions this week or worry about how many platelets are floating around in your body. You can attend family parties, Stop & Shop, and the nail salon. You get annoyed when someone drives too slow in front of you, and you honk your horn out of irritation when another driver doesn't jump when the light turns green."

My head goes on and on and on. These regular people doing regular people things make me furious inside. I let myself be angry. I'm not mad at them as much as I am at the injustice of everything. I vacillate between being grateful beyond words to my donor and medicine, as well as being angry at anyone or anything outside of my isolated world of blood cancer.

I sit on the super comfortable couch I purchased from the Facebook marketplace when Kyle and I decided to separate. I got a deal on the couch, and it's perfect. I felt weirdly empowered to make this purchase because it represented more than a piece of furniture. It represented me seeking out the simplest of stabilities. A place to sit is all I need moving forward. A place to sit, reflect, and rest in knowing that my life will be stable again. But at that moment, I don't feel stable.

I'm stalling my 30-minute walk. I hunched forward, elbows on my knees, rocking back and forth on my heels. I'm willing myself to stand up and go out into the 35-degree air. I open the door, take a sigh, start my timer, and walk.

I want this over with so badly, but my doctor says I have to do it. If I have done anything right through this process, I know I have listened to every word my doctor has said. I do not rely on Google, listen to others, or dismiss the most straightforward suggestions from medical staff. I take it in, hold it to my chest like gold, and do my best to follow the instructions. A great baker follows the recipe with precision. Cooking is less forgiving when it comes to the exactness of measurements. I'm a much better baker than a cook. I always have been.

I called a very good friend of mine on the day of diagnosis. The words spilled out of my mouth, all sloppy and messy. "It's Leukemia, it's Leukemia. What am I going to do!?" My friend's response was, "Ok. (long pause) You are in the hospital with all the right people. It's exactly where you need to be. Just listen to them."

It was a two-minute conversation, but it was exactly what I needed. I held onto those words and continued to. People are put in your life

257

for tiny, significant, and in-between moments. And some people are put in your life for a specific moment. There have been lots of specifics with my friend. Hold onto the ones who make you feel this way. They understand more about you than you realize. So humble yourself, listen to them, and know that no relationship is a mistake. It's all used—all of it.

I've been presenting on such topics as depression, fear, anxiety, de-escalation, and emotional regulation through my Social and Emotional Learning Company for the past seven years. I have poured hours upon hours into reading the latest Psychology Journal articles, checking out books from the library, and spending too much money on Amazon deliveries, where fresh pages are scribbled with notes and highlighted.

I sat in coffee shops, bookstores, and the sidelines of soccer practices, piecing together Google Slideshows for Staff Professional Development Workshops. I took my work seriously. This was important information to share with students and teachers, and I wanted it to be thorough yet attainable.

This was important information for me to understand, and it helped me better comprehend the inner workings of my teens. Even though they claim that deep breaths, self-awareness, and recognizing feelings mean nothing to them, I know they will understand someday. Actions are caught, not taught. And I'm doing my best to live in the healthiest of actions I can.

And here I am in January. Everything is gray, lonely, and hard. Quick, taunting visions of my former hospital rooms scoot through my brain like a toddler playing chase. I shudder, I avoid, I wince, and I know that at some point, I will have to revisit these visions in their entirety to heal. For now, I'm a shining example of all the content regarding depression, anxiety, fear, and PTSD that I prided myself on presenting to others.

Learning the academic and statistical portions of your studies is one thing, but it's a different ball game when you find yourself living it. The fear of daily blood count drops marks the beginning of January.

January is angry because I can't snuggle my kids or see my friends. January is riddled with anxiety about whether or not my progress will continue or if everything will come crashing down. January is depressing, and I'm wondering if anyone cares. January is the fetal position on my yoga mat, hating myself that I can't do one single push-up, and a magnesium IV drip that follows me to the bathroom.

And it's in January that I take 20 minutes to fill my weekly pillbox, only to throw it against the wall a few minutes later. All 150 pills fly through the air like pastel-colored confetti, and I spend the next 30 minutes on my hands and knees, picking every single one of them up. I crawl around, laughing and crying at the absurdity of it all.

And it feels so fucking good.

I read somewhere that January 17th is the date when, statistically, most people fail to follow through with their New Year's resolutions. I always hung onto this fact because I couldn't accept not following through with something I set my sights on.

I am not a resolution girl, a fan of them, and I do not see the need for a date on the calendar as the motivating factor to begin something. Many people may disagree with me on this way of thinking, but I come from a line of thought that holds that anything worth doing is

259

worth doing in the present. And that's where January conflicts with this mantra that has carried me through so many difficult times.

January 2023 makes me want to give up. Every single day is lonely. I should write at least ten minutes a day because I have so many ideas, but I lack the inertia even to know where to begin. I know I should look forward to Easter, summer, Thanksgiving, and Christmas this year, but I stop those visions almost as quickly as I think of them.

If I had made a resolution on January 1st to be positive and only see the best, I would have failed miserably by the 2nd. It's the first time in this mess of the past 7 months that I can't muster up one positive thought. I watch sad movies so that I will become sad. I keep the lights off when it's sunny out. I go to bed at 7 pm to finish the day.

And I became friends with depression and kind of like it. I don't have to give any emotional energy to anyone else, and I'm savvy enough to hide my sadness from the kids. And shamefully, I find myself not even wanting to see them. For no other reason than how much energy it took to pretend to be okay around them. Thoughts that used to begin with *I can't wait until I'm better so I can... to Maybe March 6th will be my last birthday.*

It's some evening in January, and I'm going through my bedtime routine. I drink eight oz. of Crystal Light, have a snack, take my medication at 7 pm, take my sleeping medication an hour later, shower, and then brush my teeth. I towel off after getting out of the shower and absentmindedly grab a second towel to wrap my hair. Out of muscle memory, I bow forward and wrap the towel around my head, remembering there was nothing to be wrapped or dried. I drop the towel, lean forward, and steady myself with one hand on each side of the sink. I can't get one single tear out. I feel so much, but I don't even know what it is. But my body knows. I look at my fingers as they turn white around the knuckles as I grip the edge of the sink. I stare into my eyes and see an 8-year-old girl full of fear, with gray circles shadowing her eyes, which were bright just a year ago. And then I see the bald head. I don't avoid it by throwing on a beanie. I look at it, and I crumble into a naked piece of flesh on the super soft Target bathroom rug that welcomes me like a security blanket. My eyes scan the tile floor of the apartment, reminding me to sweep. I feel so hideous. So unattractive. So worthless. And it's the first time in this mess that I think dying might not be so bad.

I stayed there for a long time and imagined who would come to my funeral. I guess what Kyle would say to those who stayed long enough at the funeral home to hear the Eulogy. I wondered how my parents would get through the viewing and who would carry my casket. I wondered what pictures would be put on my memory board and what restaurant everyone would go to after. I wonder if my girls would start wearing some of the clothes they always ask to borrow, or if it would be too hard. And the most complicated thought of all... who is going to absorb and hold the emotional pain for my children if their mother isn't there? I don't snap out of any of this darkness. It's depression. January sucks.

Truth 37: Hurdles

The only thing you can do is what you can do right now.

I had the fortunate yet unfortunate experience of being part of a nationally-ranked cross-country team throughout my high school sports career. My one claim to fame is that in 1995, we were the 6th-ranked team in the country. I vividly remember my coach running down the halls of our high school, excitedly shaking a newspaper copy of USA Today to celebrate our accomplishment. The miles spent on pavement, tracks, and wooded trails helped create the disciplined nature I carry today.

I say "unfortunately" because the pressures involved at this level of sport were sometimes too much. In addition to high school friend and boyfriend drama, the demands of schoolwork, and household chores, I was emotionally overwhelmed.

I was often the fifth or sixth scoring teammate in my pack of seven. In cross-country, this is an essential place on the team as the first five runners who cross the line score. The sixth and seventh runners are tiebreakers. The lower the number you end up placing, the higher the score for your team collectively. My fifth or sixth placement in races translates to being screamed at by parents and coaches in the last half mile, as I try to pass as many opponents as possible. Mentally, it was a lot. And my love for the sport was replaced with an anxious heart rate, toe on the chalk line in the grass as I waited for the gun.

As I've mentioned, people are put in our lives for a reason. Meaningful relationships are never wasted in our continued and potential growth. One of those people was my coach. We referred to him as "Mindel," his last name. I regret not calling him coach. But his role was such that he was friends with us as well as a hard ass at times when we didn't hit our 400m. split times in a workout. He knew how to balance a gaggle of 15-year-old girls crying over breakups and yelling at us in a race in a way that he knew we would understand, according to our personalities.

He handled all of us differently. We knew that and appreciated him even if we didn't have the teenage voice to express it. He annoyed us, but I'm sure we annoyed him much more. We were a small family who deeply understood the guts-to-glory theme this sport carried. And those who thought our sport looked boring or made no sense. We just rolled our eyes at comments like, "I couldn't play a sport where I wasn't chasing or throwing a ball! Running? Why would I just run?" We knew why we ran, and that was all that mattered. Ask us today as 40-somethings what our best 400 m split, mile, or 5k times were. Ask us to recall the details of a course we ran only once, and we will not fail to provide precise details. Between the summer and mid-November training months, our world was tying laces, butterflies on starting lines, and injury prevention.

It was the start of my senior year. This was my last high school season, and I was ready to be done. However, I needed to maintain the momentum as I was awarded a partial scholarship to attend college. Our first practice of this year began with a team meeting in an empty biology room after school. The front of the room featured a large, long whiteboard that spanned the wall. We sat at high-top desks where microscopes stood proudly. Mindel starts drawing

263

things on the board. He draws and writes, and continues to do so. We sit there waiting, but we're unsure where this is going. After a few minutes, he puts down the black dry-erase marker, folds his arms, and takes in what he created. He looks at us and says something along the lines of, "Girls, this season is all about hurdles." He scratched out about seven hurdles on the board, the best he could. Underneath each hurdle was a race or milestone we would strive to hit in our season to make it to states.

The first hurdle was likely a rival team, such as Saratoga or Shenendehowa. The next few hurdles were our conference race, state qualifier, State meet, and Federation meet. For some reason, this visual resonated with me. It worked well for an anxious teen like myself because I could see my season in pieces, not just one scary thought: *Coach wants us to make it to states, and what if I disappoint him or my team?* This way of thinking was addressed by allowing us to focus on only the next task ahead. To this day, I strive to apply this principle in my own life.

The truth is that we are healthier when we live simply. It means not becoming overwhelmed by big events on the horizon or changes we know we need to make. I realize that this is easier said than done. Some of us are built with this tenacity and dedication toward a goal more easily than others. But even for those for whom this comes naturally, it still works and involves staying mindful and reining yourself to the present moment when self-doubt or passiveness rears its head. Repeating to yourself daily, "I can only do what I can do right now," has been my go-to strategy to overcome the big and scary. Now is everything.

Life presents these big things, but these thoughts and roadblocks associated with them are beaten down one brick at a time with a "right now" way of thinking. We need to set goals for ourselves. Goals keep our heads in the game of life. They help us stay true to who we are and, even better, who we could be. However, these goals and whispers of things we need to change only begin when we shift our thinking.

I knew divorce was on the horizon for me about eight years ago. The thought caused unrest, panic, and a scramble to try to fix things. In my mind, divorce was not an option. That's not how I was raised, and something that would be judged by both my family and possibly my children. So, I decided to figure things out quickly because everything was falling apart rapidly. I planned getaways, bought concert tickets, put more date nights on the calendar, and started marriage counseling. I wanted to save my marriage, and Kyle did, too. But it felt like the harder we tried, the harder it became. And I became resentful toward Kyle because I didn't know if he felt as desperate as I did about our situation.

I never wanted my life to turn out like this. No one does. We don't get married expecting to get divorced 22 years later. And I get sad. I watch other couples and families on the boardwalk enjoying their family vacation. At the same time, I'm happy to have delightful memories of trips to Disney, ski trips, adventures in New York City, and our annual trip to Canada with Kyle's family. These memories blend joy, younger children, and a feeling of gratitude for having this work well for about twelve years.

But the years that followed created a sacrifice in many ways. I was at the mercy of scrambling to save an already lost marriage. I was trying to fool my children that we were okay. They could be the first ones to tell us that we weren't. They dealt with it, and I know their healthy marriage model is far from what it could have been. I regret staying in my marriage as much as I did. However, I want to believe that they will someday understand why we made the decision we did. And I will be brave and share that I was the one who initiated and walked away. I couldn't keep faking it. I couldn't keep striving toward being like other families. I was exhausted. Like an egg without a yolk. A dry shell, ready to crack with the slightest of pressure. And here, at this precipice of "what do I do?", I remember the analogy introduced to me through the concept of hurdles back in September 1998.

So, I began applying the analogy to my big life races. How was I going to beat Leukemia? Where would I be in a year? I had to push aside those big mountains and look at the next step. The next blood draw, the subsequent biopsy, the next sleepless night. How am I going to get divorced? No steady job, I need insurance, how do I do it? I was unhealthy when I looked at the big picture because it caused anxiety. How can I raise my children to be successful and, more importantly, good and kind individuals?

All these things are big questions that can crumble our silence or challenge us to grow our character. Leukemia has taught me that the more straightforward way of living is the challenging way of living. Trust the process of not knowing how things will turn out—knowing that you only have to do the next step. Eventually, you're on the mountain top, looking back and seeing all those turns in the road and valleys you hit, but somehow, you keep going. It's one at a time, one jump at a time, that gets you to the end. You don't need to know what that end is. Or maybe you do. But you can apply this principle to everyday living. Ask yourself where you are and how to better yourself in the coming moments.

Choose to live with intention. Make a promise to yourself. The only thing you can do is what you can do right now.

Truth 38: Guilt Will Destroy You

Don't let the feeling of guilt negate the truth of who you are.

I was sixteen years old. Riding horses was my safety. Flying over jumps felt like the world disappeared. My Thoroughbred and I spoke and danced in a language we only understood. He responded, I squeezed a little extra on my left calf. I used my pinky finger to manipulate the reins, and he knew exactly what his job was. It was powerful, it was unison, and it was sacred to me.

Participating in horse shows was expensive. From the class fees, transportation, and boarding, I knew my parents were giving me a good thing. And I did not take this for granted. I relished the environment, watching other riders, and studying the gates of different animals. My thoroughbred's name was "Requests A Lot," but to me, he was "Lots." He was a name well suited, as he loved attention; he was a bit goofy, but delivered stellar performances as he gracefully tackled double oxers.

I was in between classes at a local show. Lots was in his stall on the grounds with other horses, and riders proudly displayed the ribbons won on gated windows, where soft, nuzzled noses sniffed for carrots. I envied the rider's stall next to mine. She had new and neatly placed brushes organized in a fancy bin. Her saddle was covered with a custom cloth, and she had two buckets of treats for her guy. In addition, two blue ribbons and one red ribbon were displayed. My setup was nothing that compared. A bucket with a few brushes, a saddle with no cover, and no treats available. I felt sad inside that I didn't provide Lots with a more lavish exterior for his stall. And I felt worse that I had forgotten treats for him. I scanned the barn to make sure no one was around, and then I swiftly grabbed two handfuls of treats from the cool kids' territory and tucked them away in the bottom of the bin with the brushes. I took a few carrots from the bag that lay open and didn't feel an ounce of guilt as I knew how much Lots deserved these treats. I fed them to him, and it made me happy to give him some love for all he did for me in the show ring.

And then it happened. Just steps away from the barn and the quiet whinnying from horses, I felt the heaviness in my chest. I had stolen something. I had taken it without asking. I had given in to selfishness with a sneaky, desperate action. The guilt was heavy. Too heavy for a good girl who dares to do wrong because the consequence is judgment and sin. I was so upset with myself. I replayed the swiftness of my actions and condemned myself for not pausing and recognizing the implications of the emotions I might feel if I did this. I carried this feeling with me that day. I didn't win a blue or a red ribbon in the day's events. Lots and I were not in sync, not because of the heaviness of guilt, but because it got in the way of our connection.

Upon reflection, this action was not that big of a deal. I didn't rob a bank or assist with a murder. I stole a few handfuls of apple-flavored horse treats and two carrots from another rider's stall. But the guilt to follow was enough to ruin the whole reason I was there. There were no ribbons, just guilt, and it destroyed me.

Guilt isn't an emotion. It's a feeling. It's heavy and, at times, debilitating. Some of us are better than others at feeling it, but then pushing past it only until the next wave rears its head. I was not one of these people. I allowed the guilt of my actions to color the canvas of my character. I became friends with shame, guilt's sneaky cousin. And through the lies of their language, I believed I was bad. It was easier to accept the bad than to work toward self-forgiveness. It was easier to hide behind the good Christian girl script instead of coming clean about my actions. To admit my wrong to the nameless stranger who loved her horse more than mine seemed impossible. Guilt destroyed me, and I chose to make it my master.

Feeling guilty for an action is a typical and expected response. We're human. We make mistakes as swiftly as I did while snatching a few carrots. Guilt waits to reveal itself and does so immediately after we make the choice we knowingly or unknowingly made. Guilt latches onto our insecure cells and multiplies them like fuel to a flame. And if this fire is not tamed or looked at, we will become nothing but ash at the end of our lives.

Throughout my faith upbringing, a phrase repeatedly tossed about was, "God is good." A sentence a five-year-old could have come up with. And the further we grow in our character and faith, the further we distance ourselves from the simple and powerful nuggets of truth such as this one. If God is good, then why wouldn't he make us good? We are inherently all good because we are created in his image. If we were to cling to the notion that "God is guilt," our wiring would begin to interpret this feeling as true. God is good, and therefore we are good. Don't let the feeling of guilt negate the truth of who you are.

Cancer taught me to be gentle with myself. Pre-cancer, Sarah basked under the rays of guilt as I felt more comfortable with the uncomfortable than the comfort of self-love and forgiveness. I have made mistakes and regretted decisions, but I have practiced seeing myself as created in the image of God, and that image is inherently good. This is not a dismissal tactic to negate past choices. This is a moment of significant growth, where I can now view myself as an honest and imperfect human, whom Christ seeks to love and not condemn.

Our shield against guilt-ridden thoughts stemming from our actions begins with wrapping ourselves in a blanket of forgiveness and protection. Right now, actively forgive yourself for something you feel guilty about. Take a further step and mend this wound by sharing your current state of self-discovery and healing with another person who has been affected. I don't like the word "confess" as it sounds too Catholic for me. All I can see is a priest behind a dark window picking at his nails, half asleep while listening to confessions repeatedly. Instead of a confession, consider it a connection. Find a safe person, someone you trust, and ask to connect. When you do this, you feel relief, you gain perspective, and if you have found the right person, you will feel loved. And that's all any of us want in this life. We want to feel loved. Guilt will destroy you, but love will create you. We are castles in the making.

Truth 39: People Will Hurt You, Get Used to It

Through the process, I learned that I don't need outside validation because I am already overflowing with the greatness I was born with.

I've spent way too much time and energy pre-cancer worrying about what other people thought. And it wasn't until my small yet powerful internal discovery came to light. People only care about themselves. Furthermore, people do what they want to do. And on some level, most of what people do is self-serving. This isn't a bad thing; it makes sense to me. We are genetically designed to protect ourselves. It makes sense that our decisions are often made with our best interests in mind, even if it does mean hurting people along the way.

Maya Angelou is famous for saying, "When people show you who they are, believe them the first time." And even though I've returned to this quote several times, I also didn't apply it, as I made the same mistakes repeatedly and hurt myself. Before cancer, I overextended grace to people whom I thought I trusted. I cowered behind, "feeling bad" for upsetting someone or challenging their thinking. I made decisions and catered to the needs of others, without for one second considering what I wanted to do. Upon reflection, the other person often doesn't realize the sacrifices being made for their best interest. Why is that? As I've already stated, people are selfish. People only care about themselves. This way of thinking does not mean we see everyone with ill-will intentions. Instead, it's a call to be more intuitively aware of honoring your choices and walking into certain situations with an invisible shield of protection around you.

One of the reasons certain people hurt us is because they struggle with the deep-seated wounding of insecurity. Very few of us wear our wounds proudly and talk about them. That takes bravery and work, but it is always beautiful. Most of us hide our wounds as it's easier to float through life in a misty fog than a spring day's lightness. I don't judge people when they hurt me. I realize that often, they don't even know they are hurting me. I actively decide to return to the understanding that they are responding to their shit and not mine.

Before cancer, I gave too much energy to people and situations that didn't serve me best. And, sounding completely selfish, I am the most important. If I don't recognize my value and make choices based on what serves my overall well-being, I am doing a disservice to myself and others. What does it mean? It means that others will not be getting the best version of me.

Consider this scenario. A good friend who often invites you to dinner or happy hour drinks plans an event without considering that you might want to come. You see a social media post with happy selfies and half-sipped wine glasses. Pre-cancer, Sarah would have cringed, a knot in my stomach, suffocated anger, and *what's wrong with me?* internal language. However, I now embrace these opportunities to study how I respond, and after a while, it starts to feel fun because it becomes incredibly invigorating and deepens my self-worth. I learned through the process that I don't need outside validation because I am overflowing with the greatness I was already born with.

273

In the past, I would question what I had done wrong not to be invited. I would have ignored the friend and quietly sulked. Instead, I ask how the recent night out was in my newly discovered power. I watch the other person squirm, unsure of how to handle my boldness in tackling the elephant in the room head-on. And I like living this way now.

The opinions of others should never matter to you. It's about them, not you. Judgments from others about your choices are mostly made because those people don't have the tools to look at their hard stuff. However, people categorize you as something that should not concern you. Their invalid responses to who you are as a whole person are not for them to judge; it's for you to protect.

A good friend once introduced the idea of the invisible shield of protection. I have applied this practice through phone calls, face-to-face conversations, and parent-teacher conferences. It's a straightforward exercise. When walking into or finding yourself in a situation where your energy might be challenged, damaged, or drained, imagine creating an invisible and transparent shield of protection. To take this visual a step further, imagine bouncing the energy tossed your way to bounce back onto them. In this mindset, you are protected; the most remarkable thing is that your body feels this protection. It's like walking in a rainstorm, getting drenched and pelted on your cheeks with raindrops, and then discovering someone runs up alongside you and holds an umbrella over your head. Your body melts into this means of protection because you are mentally deciding to protect. Your cellular self responds with ease, rather than being stressed and ready to react. It's a beautiful process. When you honor your body, you are choosing to celebrate yourself.

Lastly, people crave reactions. And the best reactions are the ones where we are made to feel inferior, and they are made to feel powerful. Often, this is done subconsciously by the other person involved. Again, this is about their wounding and does not reflect how they might think of you. Don't get angry with the other person. Instead, practice the opposite. Send love and understanding, knowing they have a lot of work to do. Making you feel bad or left out makes them feel important. And they want to feel important because insecurity rears its ugly head at the most unsuspected times. Consider these moments a blessing in disguise because this is the Universe's way of weeding out the people you don't need in your life.

As I will declare over and over again, find your people. And even if you feel like you've found your people, challenge yourself to remain curious about it. Have you *really* found your people? I apply two simple questions to the people I associate with. Do I want to associate myself with this person or group? Do they value my character and self-growth? These are yes or no questions. If you are vulnerable and brave enough, accept the first answer that feels right. Not what you think you should feel. Listen to what your body is telling you. If I had practiced this principle before cancer, I would have had a lot less hurt and a lot more self-respect.

The bottom line is that accepting that people will hurt you is simple. Your body knows who you should be associating yourself with. It will celebrate your growth when you make the right people choices and open the floodgates for more like-minded gemstones to be added to your collection of beautiful beings. In addition, accept that most don't mean to hurt; they don't know how to communicate and connect. This is not you; this is them. The most beautiful thing you can do for another human in these situations is to love them. That's all anyone ever wants to feel. "But the greatest of these is love " (1 Corinthians 13:13).

Truth 40: Protect and Celebrate Your Gift

When we challenge our inner critic, our body does the most fantastic thing: our body celebrates you through unforeseen opportunities and increased self-esteem.

This truth may not resonate with everyone, but if you find it relatable, trust me, it's important.

I was born intuitive. I have vivid memories from my childhood of understanding another's language without a single word being spoken. It was frustrating because I had this sixth sense that I thought everyone else had, too. But they didn't. The harder I tried to ignore its whispers and utterances, the more prominent it became. And at some point in my mid-teens, I understood that this was possibly a gift, not a curse. Intuition came in dreams or a sense of something bad happening, only to find my presumption validated. So, I kept it a secret to protect its power and my own.

Reading energy is like reading a book. The words are presented, you read them, and then you learn. Energy reading is very similar. The individual is presented, you feel them, and then you are informed. If you relate to this, you know. If you often feel a sense of knowing before the outcome or sensing before admission, you know.

The ability to read energy in another individual or environment is a gift. But to know this with humble gratefulness to your creator. It's not granted to everyone freely because it's a hard lot to carry through life, and frankly, if we were all energy readers, the world might as well explode because of the spot-on intuitions we have.

Before cancer, I was very open with others about my feelings or ideas of uncertainties when it came to other people. Friends would count on me for advice or just a listening ear. I took it all in. I knew the answers, but I didn't give them freely, as most of the time, it made me feel superior, and my power scared me. I kept it hidden, and I kept my power quiet. To be clear, I'm not an empath, and I don't like that title. It presents an energy that is better than or special, separating one human being from another. Those who proudly proclaim themselves as empaths are doing so for their own gain, not for the benefit of others. It makes others feel less, and that's not how we should live. We should be connecting, not separating.

Understanding and feeling energy are different. It comes over you at the most unsuspected times and when you need it the most. It helps to guide, protect, and expect respect simultaneously. There have been many times I have chosen to ignore that deep gut, slight pain in my chest feeling. My body knew, but my mind decided to ignore it. The result of my choices was often sloppy and never supportive of providing the good things in life. And before cancer, I didn't give my gift the respect it deserved. But yet, it stuck around with my stubborn head.

I will no longer live this way. As frustrating as intuitions present themselves each day, I will honor and support this source. My body knew from day one of my diagnosis that I would be okay. When my teenage girls showed up to my hospital room after a day of surfing, sand still stuck between their toes, they tried to look brave. But when you know a human since the day they were born, you understand their mannerisms to a point of perfection. Mini billboards flashing the word fear were seen in their eyes. They did their best to show bravery. Their energy pleaded for their mom, but they protected what they didn't want to say. The idea of losing their mother was a possibility for them. But not for me. This was the only time they saw me during my 49-day stay. Day six, hooked up to machines, beeping, a mix between gray and yellow skin tone, and covered in bruises. I looked at them in the eyes, always in the eyes, and said, "Girls, I'm going to be okay. This is all going to be okay." My body and energy knew; they took that and trusted me. I was right. And they felt a bit more at ease.

We all have gifts. Some of us keep them hidden, while others celebrate them. When we keep them hidden, we are doing the Universe a disservice as we can't use it to its fullest potential. We feel ill-equipped, inadequate, or unworthy of what we might be good at.

Understanding that you are good at something is the start. I am confident that most of us walk around in fear and self-doubt. Over comparing, over-posting a near-perfect life on Facebook, and questioning why we aren't successful. And the choice is ours. We either stay stuck in the hamster wheel of lies or step off and bravely take the next right step. When we challenge our inner critic, our body does the most fantastic thing: our body celebrates you through unforeseen opportunities and increased self-esteem. This is all because God "has created you for such a time as this" (Esther 4:14).

Your place in this world matters as much as the next person. It's not to tell others how to use their power; it's for you to discover your own. Do not let the successes of others diminish your vision of success. They are on their journey, and you are on yours. And though both journeys are important, yours is more important. This is not a selfish way of thinking; it's a necessary way of thinking. You will find that when you shift into the mindset of 'I am powerful, worthy, and separate from others,' you begin to discover how the Universe will use your gift in magical ways.

One of my great loves is teaching kids yoga. We dance, balance, play games, and practice meditation in ways that allow us to connect. They are a clear source of understanding the world around them. We don't respect their abilities to know things that we do not know. And we don't give them the outlets to be curious about who they are. They are closer to the source of life, the womb. They come into the world as pure and, over time, are disappointed as their big souls become smaller and smaller due to the negative influences of the world around them. Every once in a while, I come across a student or child who gets it and has not yet experienced the disappointment of what they thought life could offer, only to discover it doesn't.

For the sake of anonymity, I will refer to this yoga student as Lucy. Lucy faithfully attended class, and from the very first day, she fell in love with it. She did not participate in a sports team, didn't play a musical instrument, and art wasn't her thing either. She didn't fit the typical 13-year-old girl's mold. She didn't swoon over Taylor Swift and didn't wear white van slip-on shoes like all her other friends. She was quiet, and I liked her. I liked her because she knew she was different and owned it. Her hair was long and untamed. She was slightly overweight and self-conscious, often wearing a large, oversized t-shirt to every yoga class. The theme of one specific class centered on affirmations and discovering that we can change our mindset by how we speak to ourselves.

Each student was to write an affirmation on a large poster board. We would then recite all of them as a group. I told them to write the first affirmation that came to them and not to overthink it. I was curious; Lucy was the first to write her affirmation on the board.

Once all ten students had completed their affirmations, most related their affirmations to milk and honey ideas. "I am great, I am awesome, I am happy, I am strong, I am amazing." In large print in the center of the board, as if owning the board and putting the others in a backseat, read, "I am worthy." I take a deep breath and look at her. She sits cross-legged, twirling her hair, unaware of the power of her affirmation. We talked about all the affirmations, and I saved hers for last. "Lucy, what does it mean to feel worthy?"

Her response. "It means that I deserve good things."

Friends, good things come to those who believe they are worthy and brave enough to take the next step into their gift. Let's be more like Lucy.

Truth 41: Extend Grace

When the grace of others is offered sparingly, the molecules of self-confidence dwindle over time.

I love words. I always have. And I find it clever that some words sound like their meanings. For me, the word "grace" is one of those words. It floats off your tongue like a slender ballerina in a pirouette. It feels light, bright, and magical. However, it also carries a heavy responsibility. As presented in scripture, "Let us then with confidence draw near to the throne of grace, that we may receive mercy and find grace to help in time of need " (Hebrews 4:16)

Daily, we are tempted by choices that are not good for ourselves or others. We make choices that hurt others. We are selfish, greedy, and human in every sense. We make mistakes and sometimes carry the guilt associated with them for years. This is not healthy. The truth of extending grace challenges us to forgive ourselves and extend grace to those who are hard to forgive. And as Christ extends grace to us, we are called to do the same for others. Ultimately, our bodies become more transparent as we practice more grace.

I fell in love with studying Psychology in college. I was an education major, as my dad advised me to pursue a degree that I could apply immediately upon graduation. He was right. However, the classes I looked forward to the most were Child Psychology, Abnormal Psychology, and Cognitive Psychology. The ideas were fascinating, and the greats who paved the way, like Freud, Bandura, Piaget, and Maslow, were my heroes. Their theories and discoveries were fascinating. I gravitated to the different teaching styles of my professors. Still, I was drawn to one over the others because of his demeanor and willingness to actively practice extending grace to his students.

Mr. Stegan was a gentle man who wore a perfectly sculpted comb-over and quietly delivered his teaching. He wasn't ruffled if a student walked in ten minutes late to class; he welcomed students into his office and stayed after class to dive deeper into a topic if I was interested. His teaching style wasn't everyone's cup of tea, but for me, he gained my respect because he saw his students as human and early twenty-somethings who were trying to figure out life and undoubtedly going to make mistakes along the way.

This is where I learned what it meant to extend grace in the most basic ways. And forever, I will remember how this approach made me feel. No other professor followed suit, so I don't know how the others influenced my thinking. One of my favorite authors, Maya Angelou, stated, "I've learned that people will forget what you said, people will forget what you did, but people will never forget how you made them feel."

Mr. Stegan was known for his grace philosophy regarding the due dates for his assignments. I quickly noticed that other professors in the department rolled their eyes at this practice, but as students, we readily adopted it. He happily accepted assignments handed in on the specific due date, but he offered the next step of "grace" to hand in two days later. If that deadline didn't work, he extended "extra grace" for two days beyond the grace period.

Lastly, "mega grace" was given one week after the initial due date. At the time, I thought Mr. Stegan was giving us a break on the assignment due dates. Upon reflection, he was doing much more. He was modeling to us how it felt to have grace extended. We could miss a due date without shame, knowing we had a few extra days. Without judgment, we could miss the next due date and put ourselves at ease with another few days. For him, it wasn't a tactic to cut us some slack. It held a greater purpose. As one of my favorite quotes reads, "Actions are caught, not taught." Through one professor's modeling of extending grace, I learned what it felt like to be on the receiving end. This, in turn, taught me the importance of extending grace to others to cultivate relationships and, most importantly, heal our self-wounding.

Our bodies crave acceptance to maintain emotional health. We want to feel confident and assured that we are essential. When others refuse to forgive or extend a second chance, we quickly take this to heart, and our character is colored, but not with pretty colors. It's a tough pill to swallow, especially if we've been fed these pills in our upbringing.

When the grace of others is offered sparingly, the molecules of self-confidence dwindle over time. Just as much as we crave the grace provided through the forgiveness of others, we must also acknowledge our actions in offering grace to those who have hurt us. The result is deeper relationships and a newly discovered vulnerability landscape between two people. In this way of thinking, the veils of perfection are lowered, and the action of extending grace brings two people closer.

One of the simplest lessons that Leukemia has taught me is that wasting time on petty troubles in relationships is not worth our precious energy. I have learned that I am the keeper of my sacred energy—the energy of pure cells celebrating each day without being infected with animosity. Walking a tightrope of near death, I have come to value forgiveness over success. This is only experienced through receiving grace, but more importantly, giving it.

The conflict with extending grace is that often, we are the ones who need it the most. We can practice extending to others, but when it comes to ourselves, we are hesitant and tread lightly, as we don't think we deserve it. I'll always wonder why we are our own worst critics. If we are given one body to keep healthy physically, why do we struggle so much to maintain our emotional well-being? The only answer I have is that we don't deem ourselves worthy. We don't see ourselves as humans who make mistakes. Instead of accepting that mistakes are learning opportunities in disguise, we attach to them. Over time, the guilt of our actions builds a wall that prevents us from receiving the grace our bodies so desperately crave.

The verse stated in Hebrews urges us to approach the throne with confidence. The verse doesn't call one to approach the throne in your current state. It's a call to walk boldly and with strength, knowing that you are just as deserving as the next to receive the grace you might not believe you are worthy of. Sprinkling doses of grace on actions, present or past, that you are ashamed of might not erase your guilt, but it will begin to build your soul character.

My sweet mom was the most significant influencer in my relationship with Christ. She saw Him as her father, her husband, and the first to have a conversation with every morning. She would sit at our kitchen table every morning with a coffee cup, a bible open, and cozy in her silky, flower-patterned robe. She woke to the scriptures, and they spoke to her. She once explained grace through a word picture I will forever cling to. "Imagine, Sarah, that grace is always floating above you. And all you have to do is reach up and take a handful whenever you need it." And that's just it. Grace is offered freely, just hovering above us, accessible and plenty. Just be sure you accept that grace with all the confidence you can muster because you, my darling, are worth more than all the stars in the sky.

Truth 42: Death Does Not Hold You

If we turn our cheek and make death and grief our new identity, we limit our potential to grow and to start receiving the good things that the Universe has for us.

I sank deeply into the cushions of my forest-green microfiber couch. A purchase I was proud of, and one that seemed to complete our living room. I chose it for its durability against baby spit-up and toddler messes. It was always just a couch to sit on and enjoy a movie or to be destroyed to create crooked foundations for Saturday afternoon forts. But in that moment, this couch became my cave of isolation, depression, and anger.

I say goodbye to Kyle as he leaves for work, and I pack lunches and homework folders to send the kids to school. When all humans are out of the house, I become friends with the darkness by making it darker. I pull the shades, turn off the lights, and silence my phone. I stay in my pajamas for the day and fall into the couch. The room is dark, the TV is on, and there are no people. It feels like a high. A high defined by death where the darker it became, the more I could feel the pain. I was an addict, and my drug of choice was seeing how far down the path of pain I could get. My goal was not to feel anything at all.

Just a few days prior, I gave birth to a tiny, lifeless baby boy. His name was Magnus William, Max for short. A strong name, as it was taken after his maternal grandfathers. He slipped through me. We said goodbye briefly when we greeted each other with a touch and a shared energy as his body slid limply from mine. Birthing unto death is heavy. Birthing unto life is light. Birthing unto death feels like death itself. Birthing unto life creates new life. I made death my friend; I welcomed it in and allowed it to take over every thought and every action, and very slowly, I became entangled in its grasp. I wanted my baby boy. It was all unfair. No one understood the pain. No one but me. To feel a life within you, tiny feet kicking, squirmy body turning, to feel a void. To feel a lifeless lump of soul energy slip through with ease is a feeling etched like a fossil in the cellular structure of my soul.

I tried to put on a brave face when people were around. I volunteered at school for the kids' events. I kept up with the meals and the housework. I hid behind a fake smile when people offered continued condolences. I kept it all tucked neatly away for only me to worry about. I didn't want to be a bother to anyone, and quite frankly, I also didn't want to share my pain with them because that was for me and my baby to have to ourselves.

I was selfish with my pain. I didn't talk about it, work on it, and refused to share it. It was mine. Death was mine. Darkness was mine, and it felt so good. The hands of death gripped tightly and pulled me away from the tiny other hands that wanted their mommy. I became resentful of my younger children. Their needs seemed so much needier. Their behavior seemed to escalate after the loss, and I retaliated with discipline rather than love. I was a thunderstorm of agony, grief, and anger hiding behind a 30-something stay-at-home mom who was trying to keep breathing.

Eventually, I took baby steps toward working through the pain of the loss—therapy appointments, writing, and processing through tears and remembrances of this ache in my life. I came up with a sweet ritual of holding his blanket against my cheeks as it absorbed the tears while taking in the intricacies of his stamped footprints, which the hospital sent home. I do this every year on his birthday.

Over time, I learned that I had power over death and that it was no longer welcome to have control over me. I welcomed the heaviness, darkness, and ache but did not feed it this time. I sat in it and allowed it to stay for a bit. It was no longer welcome to have a hold on me. I was the one in charge. I spoke to it. I put death in its place and practiced a clever tactic of beginning to look at Max's death as a form of beauty in disguise. It wasn't until many years later that I realized Max was a sacrifice to elevate me to a higher place in my life and in my soul as a woman and a mother. I owe it to my sweet baby boy for allowing opportunities and growth that would have never been there if we hadn't parted ways on January 14th, 2013.

We must honor death and sink into the grief, the tears, and all the stages associated. However, we must also be attuned when losing ourselves to the sneaky thorns of grief. If we turn our cheek and make death and grief our new identity, we limit our potential to grow and to start receiving the good things that the Universe has for us. Our cells need to grieve the loss. We are doing our bodies a disservice if we don't mourn the loss. However, if we get too comfortable in our grief, we then begin clinging to it as a safety. We take on this grief as our new identity. And that's how I responded when I watched my nurse carry my lifeless baby boy in a hand-knit, tan hospital blanket out of my delivery room. I and darkness became friends, and I wouldn't share my friend with anyone. I didn't share because I knew that if I tried, the other person wouldn't feel the pain as hard as I was. And why did I need to talk about it if they couldn't feel it?

I have learned that honoring my body comes not only in the form of a healthy way of living, wholesome relationships, and making good choices. It also involves self-awareness of when I am being pulled in a direction that isn't good for me. It consists of letting down the shield of pride when another tries to help me move out of my comfort zone. There is no need to be a rockstar in hiding your pain when going through something that looks like a mountain not meant for you to climb. You are only crippling your life source reserves if you think you can handle it all on your own.

One of the reasons I love scripture is that it presents vivid word pictures. Children are experts at memorizing scripture because the words create a picture or a story, and the brain cements the nugget of truth. At least, that's how it worked for me. This is one of those verses. "Weeping may endure for an evening, but joy comes in the morning." (Psalm 30:5). I am not minimizing our grief to endure for the literal meaning of an evening. Instead, I'm encouraging that this grief, this darkness, this deep well of hurt doesn't last forever. You acknowledge it there, but then you actively practice healthy principles to help yourself live and grow through it. Grief can be part of you, but not the whole of you. Turn the perspective a bit. What if grief helped you become the whole person you were meant to be? Just as we welcome fear, we also welcome grief. We must ride the wave of where it takes us and be okay knowing that we don't have to make it our identity. It is part of us, but it is not all of us.

Losing my baby boy was one of the most potent tastes of death I have yet to experience. I know there will be many more of these tastes as I say goodbye to some I love the most. But I've learned that clinging to death only takes away from my own life. Christ designed us to live fully and with joy. Sadness, heartache, disappointment, and all of the other hard things will always rear their head, but the joy that follows in the morning is a sweet taste of understanding how beautiful this life is.

Max's Lullaby

My dear Magnus William,
How my womb it does grieve.
But the joy of carrying you, that will never leave.
I look forward to meeting you,
just beyond those great gates.
Oh, my dear Magnus William, please always wait.

February 2023: Who Am I?

Life still feels super slow and laborious. I march forward daily with my eyes set on March 1st— day 100. Tiny wisps of newborn-like hair are starting to make their debut, making me happy. My appetite started to kick, but none of the foods I liked appealed to me. Before my transplant, I was an avid coffee drinker every morning, and the thought of coffee now makes me cringe. I was raised on red sauce, and now it seems boring. Sweets were never my thing. I always ate the obligatory piece of birthday cake at a party, as you NEVER skip a piece of cake on someone's birthday. That's one of the simplest ways you can celebrate them. I want Swedish fish, chocolate cupcakes, and Boston Cream Donuts.

I've read that others have experienced changes in their tastes after transplant. I took this information with a grain of salt and a shrug of my shoulders. I never expected that something as finite as taste could be altered. I like to think that my donor has a sweet tooth, which might be one of the first questions I ask him when we meet.

February has always been an annoying month for me. It holds onto the cold and offers little to look forward to. Other than its ending and Spring's beginning. My irritation stems from what I have always considered the most ridiculous holiday. As a child, I didn't look forward to Valentine's Day parties in the classroom because there was too much pressure. Little girls with hearts too big for their bodies would compare Pretty Pony Valentines to see who received the better one from the classroom crush. Middle school lunchroom fundraisers involving carnation sales were an in-your-face reminder of who meant something to someone and who didn't. My best friend would casually accept five carnations from 5 different boys in the class. The girls who were lucky enough to be bought a .50 carnation carried them around from class to class as a symbol of popularity and recognition. I was never one of those girls. I wanted to be, but was also conflicted because I didn't want to be. I was sad, jealous, and envious, but mostly, I was annoyed. Why could one day hold such emotional weight that could build up or destroy a 14-year-old girl's sense of self-worth? And to this day, carnations make absolutely no sense to me. They are the fall-back flowers.

If I see a man walking out of the food store with a bouquet of carnations for his wife, I secretly scorn him. He went the cheap route. He could have spent seven more dollars for an upgrade to roses, but the truth is that he doesn't care about whatever occasion it is. If he did, he would invest in the details. Carnations are bought out of obligation, and the woman knows that. But she stuffs down her disappointment and accepts the half-hearted gesture.

You may be judging my opinion on this, and that's okay. But women must understand that their self-worth far exceeds the Pretty Pink Pony Valentine's. Accepting the cheaper petals with little fragrance is self-limiting. Wait for the roses, or better yet, your favorite flower. Mine are sunflowers.

Aside from dealing with my natural annoyance of February's return each year, this month out of the past eight months of this hell has thrown me for the biggest loop. I'm out of treatment, in remission, recovering, getting stronger, and finally home. All these things would lead one to think that this was a good month for me. It was not. It was not a good month because I didn't know who "me" was. My body no longer carried Leukemia, but I felt like I *was* Leukemia.

293

And this thought, this false embodiment of something that wasn't there, defined every thought, movement, and decision I made. I didn't know how to be "Yoga Sarah," "Mom Sarah," or "Friend Sarah." I tried reading books and articles about things that would have been super interesting to me before this mess. I tried journaling, puzzles, and working out in my basement. Nothing felt the same. It all felt forced. I felt like the Universe was messing with me and teasing me.

Here you are, thinking you're better. Look at you trying to move past this beast. You no longer even know who you are. You will always be the cancer mom in town. You will never have what you had before. You think you beat cancer, but clearly, it's still bigger than you since you can't figure out who you are anymore.

The conflict and the truth in all this is that I didn't know who I was because I knew intuitively that I would never be that person again. The person I was before the cancer is gone now. She's the one who said yes to everyone except herself. She's the one who chose the crumbs instead of the entire meal. She's the one who took the burdens of her teenagers' bad decisions as a reflection of her character and not theirs. She's the one who worked four jobs because she was too fearful to let go of the other half of a relationship that didn't provide enough. She's the one who chose to look in a mirror and see imperfection rather than beauty, grace, and strength. She's the one who decided not to be true to herself and her needs.

There is one word in the human language I could do without, mainly because, 90% of the time, it is used out of context, and people fall into the habit of melting it into conversation without thinking about it. "I literally died. I'm literally starving. I'm literally going to explode."

It drives me nuts, but I swallow my pride and continue conversations with people who use the word "literally" to create mini shock-and-awe as they accompany it with hand gestures. However, in my current situation, I'm okay with saying that I'm *literally* starting life from scratch. I'm a newborn baby with a new immune system, new DNA, zero immunizations, and an opportunity to re-create a life opposite to the one I've lived for 44 years. And this thought is very exciting to me. I've had hours and hours of alone time in hospital beds to think about this idea. I bounce back and forth between 'This is such an awesome gift!' and 'What happens if I screw up worse the second time around in this chance of life?'

And that's how I see this whole thing. I'm given a second chance. The second half of life is to stand stronger, say no more often, say yes to myself, not hide behind three glasses of wine at night, and make spontaneous bad decisions on a weekend night out with my girlfriends. Because of it, I'm given a second chance to allow my teenagers to see me as honest, broken, and beautiful. But things are different now. I cry in front of them and share my frustrations. I hold 8-year-olds having tantrums while I silently scold myself for not doing this more when my teenagers were this age. I let my teens know that I didn't expect to have a broken family and that it makes me sad not to have given them the life they thought they would have. I've lived in fear, lies, and "shoulds" for 44 years. I embodied this without even knowing it.

The real truth is that the body knows. You don't have to tell it what it needs to know because it's the ultimate teacher. It's whether or not we pause to listen to it. I ignored this teacher for my entire life. Falling into behavior patterns that don't challenge or change you is easier.

Change is uncomfortable and often requires us to be vulnerable. Not just vulnerable to ourselves but to others. I ignored the moments to be "real." I faked it. I made it look like roses on the outside while I was slowly wilting on the inside. My body was rejecting me as I was not honoring all it had done for me. My physical body earned me a running scholarship for college. My physical body has given birth to six beautiful children. One that I look forward to meeting someday.

My body produces ideas, thoughts, and emotions that I can put into words and put on paper. And it was this physical body that I took for granted. I selfishly thought it would tag along and keep up with the unhealthy choices I was making. The body knows. And my body knew that for me to live my most prosperous life, it had to slowly start to die, for me to begin to live again.

February gives way to March through long, dark, dull days, with many visits to Hope Tower. In a backward way, I looked forward to my bi-weekly appointments. I cried one morning on the way to an appointment because I felt pathetic as I looked forward to seeing my friends. The nurses and doctors have now been with me for 8 months. I am familiar with their families, goals, and recent vacations. They have never treated me like someone with blood cancer who had no hope. They always made me feel like a human being and alive. Greeted me with a smile, asking about my kids and how I felt emotionally.

Blood test results and chemistry numbers came later in the appointment, but only after I was seen as a person first. Through our connection, I realized I had also begun to see myself as a human being. They made me feel important; they made me feel as though I mattered, and they made me feel loved. And it's possible that the root of those tears during that one drive came from me beginning to understand that I mattered. Throughout my life, I have viewed others as the ones who mattered. *What can I do for her? What does he need? Where can I help? She needs support. That family needs a meal.* I bypassed the truth that I might be the one who needed those things, and often more than just one at a time. Drip by drip, my well became dry. It became so dry that it forgot its purpose was to hold water.

So I lived in this dryness and rejected any buckets of water, feeling unworthy enough to receive them.

Eventually, I started to receive water from those around me, and I began to recognize their actions as genuine in their willingness to help. This help comes in the form of meals, Christmas gifts for the kids, gift cards, medicine pick-ups at the pharmacy, play-dates for my kids, and surprising my family with a fully decorated house for Christmas. And through these acts of kindness, I realized that one theme carried the most weight.

Those who you would expect to support you the most seemed to retreat. And the ones least expected to support my family came through in deep ways. This awareness didn't bother me. Instead, it encouraged me to recognize the sincere goodness in people. I only knew some of these bucket-fillers through short conversations, quick emails, or a "hello" in the produce section of Stop n' Shop. Some of them were friends of my close friends. And not once did I question why some friends retreated or became silent. I was self-aware enough to understand that each person handles emotions in their own capacity. Blood cancer is heavy. The outcome is often bleak. So what is there to say to the one moving through the muddy waters of uncertainty? Not a whole lot. It can be uncomfortable; it can bring up past hurt in losing someone they had loved, and it can induce fear related to *What if it was me with this diagnosis?*

I love my mom. So much. I love her for an infinite number of reasons. But if I were to put all these reasons in a colander and sift out the most important reason, it would be her selfless servant heart toward others. Throughout my life, I watched her make apple pies for a neighbor who had just had surgery; she also volunteered her time at my grandmother's nursing home and led Bible studies. She made meals for people; she took in those who didn't have a place to go for holidays, and hosted big team parties for cross-country, softball, and track at our home. She held space for women moving through divorce and broken marriages. She led bible studies in her home and volunteered as a Youth for Christ teen leader. She listened with empathy, and she felt deeply. Those who cross her path know that they are immediately accepted and loved. As my oldest son once said, "Mom, I think MeMe is the nicest human on the planet."

My mother continues to live her life as "the church." She embodies the awareness that church doesn't just mean Sunday services at 9 am. It doesn't have to mean tithing, Attending Women's retreats, or volunteering for Sunday School. My mother modeled to me that to live as the church meant to see the broken and hold them. It meant seeing the lonely and taking them in, or simply offering them a hug. It is intended to provide nourishment for the tired or to aid in recovery. It meant reaching out consistently to those who had battled illness for lengthy periods.

It has been through my journey with blood cancer that my church was the people I least expected to have come through and love me. Although full of love, my hometown church did not support our family in the ways I had hoped. A bouquet and a phone call from a church leader were the only two means of support. There was no meal chain (not that I needed another!). There was no checking in on our kids to see how this was affecting them; there were no offers to help, and there was no house visit or hospital visit from a pastor or assistant pastor offering support and prayer.

Was I hurt? Yes. Did it inform me who the church was? Yes. Who is the church? Those who walk in love just as Christ did. It's nothing extravagant. It's nothing that needs to be noticed. It's simple. It's just one human loving another human. And when the body of Christ disappoints you as a collective group of people professing outreach to others, it's okay to smile and look forward.

As Mr. Rogers is known to say, "Always look for the helpers."

I had lots of helpers. Most of these helpers were strangers, but to me, they were "The Church." And maybe most of my helpers weren't faithful attendees at 9 am Church services, or who faithfully tithed 10% each week. But my helpers were real people who embodied Christ in their way.

Look beyond the brick-and-mortar for your church. Be the church to the mom in town who looks tired. Be the church to your neighbor who seems to have nothing nice to say to you...ever. Be the church to the checkout lady at Walmart, who barely looks at you. Just smile. Be the church by saying 'good morning' and 'thank you' to the strangers you encounter daily. Every human in the world wants to be seen. Be the one to see them, even just through a smile.

Truth 43: Validation is Overrated

Seeking validation creates a habit of jumping from one high to another, constantly seeking approval and accolades from any source available.

I knew I wouldn't be picked for the Junior Prom Court. But still, like every other 16-year-old girl wearing puffy sleeves in my vicinity, I was holding onto a sliver of hope. The status came with wearing the cheap gold tiara that the prom committee bought from the party store. I wondered if anyone else had nominated my name in the sparkly pink ballot box on a makeshift podium in our high school hallway just days prior. I was annoyed by my need for accolades, which I realized even back then was artificial and silly.

Moms show up outside the prom venue doors. They are huddled in the giddy hallway, waiting with their 10 ml. cameras to take pictures of the prom King and Queen announcement. And just as they wished they had been picked as the queen 20 years earlier, they hoped their daughter would shine in the spotlight that night.

There I was, in my purple prom dress, heart beating faster and trying to will something that I knew meant nothing, but I wanted it anyway. The king and queen are announced, and it's no surprise as they are the classic high school jock and a flakey blonde who was used to having things handed to them. I rolled my eyes and immediately shamed myself for investing an ounce of emotional energy into this tradition, when just seconds before the announcement, I had wanted to wear the plastic crown more than anyone in the room. And it was here that I discovered what it meant to crave outside validation.

Everyone wants a gold star. Everyone wants a medal, even if it's just a symbol of participation. The more we crave the need to be seen, the less important we feel on the inside. And half the time, we have no idea why we crave outside validation from strangers. We are so accustomed to not being curious about the iceberg below the surface that we walk through life, becoming accustomed to living in the only way we are conditioned to live. And that place is in our heads and not in our hearts. Being validated and doted on by others feels good. We feel important and like we matter. But this feeling is fleeting and not permanent. Seeking validation creates a habit of jumping from one high to another, constantly seeking approval and accolades from any source available.

I've lived the majority of my life in this space. I'm a bit ashamed of it now, but I have come out stronger for the discoveries I have made post my cancer journey. I was the mom of toddlers who sought out the perfect apple streusel crumb cake recipe on Pinterest to bring to a church bible study. I didn't want to make it. I was tired and barely had the time with youngsters clinging to me and losing their binkies. But I made the cake because it meant I would get statements of approval from people who were somewhat superficial in my life. I stepped to the plate and volunteered for committees that, behind closed doors, I resented, yet did to fuel my selfish and insecure self.

In my later years, I grew a business that I believed in, but one that ultimately led me to seek as many presentations as possible to be seen, rather than make a change. Standing in front of a few hundred educator professionals made me feel powerful. There I was, at a podium, with a presentation behind me that had taken weeks of research. Most of the crowd didn't want to be there, but I was okay with that. It was stipulated in their contract that they would participate in professional development day workshops. I wanted to be there, and as much as I believed I was doing this for them, I was also doing it for myself. I felt a slight sense of superiority and control. I loved watching people frantically take notes based on my words and the research I unveiled. I craved discussions with participants after the presentation because it meant that I had something to give them that they couldn't find anywhere else. This made me feel like someone.

My vision of bringing social and emotional learning practices to school districts didn't start like this. It started softly and humbly. I allowed opportunities to come and didn't seek out new contracts. My intentions were pure, and I began to see that, over time, I had something special. I was proud of myself. But as with most humble beginnings, the middle part starts founding itself on pride. That's exactly the place I found myself in. Pride. Seeking out the selfish gain of approval from others. I have now concluded that I craved this because, underneath the layers of a competent, powerful businesswoman, was a seven-year-old little girl who rarely received the approval she desperately hoped for.

Reflecting on the 44 years of life I had lived until my diagnosis, I realize it was defined by seeking out the plastic crowns, gold stars, awards, and the feeling of being needed and wanted. The irony is that the energy it took to keep this all up slowly depleted what I needed to survive. My energy and self-esteem were dwindling on a cellular level. My poor body was screaming at me to believe that I was already enough. But the louder it became, the more I snuffed it out. My body then began only to whisper that I was enough. Eventually, my body became silent and threw the white flag of surrender. As ugly as leukemia is, it is also redeemed through the beauty of its lessons. Leukemia is responsible for saying, "Sarah, you are worthy to be alive because you, my darling, are just naturally worthy." And that's all it is. A knowing and an embodiment of believing that we are worthy in our own space, separate from the prom court.

I now live intentionally and mindfully each day, considering what I truly need. Not what others need and certainly not what they need from me. Sometimes, I find myself seeking cheap crowns, but I'm more able to reflect on what I'm doing. One of the ways I've become better at this practice is by watching how others live. The mom who volunteers at school, makes the perfect cupcakes, and has the best-decorated house at Halloween is likely the most insecure. I know this because that mom was me for far too many years. All that striving equates to your body dipping into the reserves of what is barely left. You go to bed tired and resentful of others, and think about what you can do next to fuel your need for approval.

Begin implementing a new philosophy regarding celebrating who you are and how you fit into this world. Start by believing that you are loved simply because of your place in this world. Your doings should be only what feels right and aligns with your intentions. As soon as you do something that feels forced or contrived, this is the clue that you are not doing it for the right purpose. If attuned, you will become adept at recognizing when you are making choices based on the approval of others rather than yourself. The energy spent seeking approval is not worth the risk of receiving one minute of accolades from a friend who says, "Wow, this crumb cake is

303

amazing! How do you find the time to bake with three toddlers at home?" Ahh, it feels lovely to receive a compliment, and then, poof, the feeling is gone. A momentary high was replaced with an empty feeling of what I could do next to get some feel-good feedback. It's a cycle of approval that keeps repeating unless you stop it in its tracks, take a stand, and challenge it.

Now, I live wearing a crown I created and designed, and can add to whenever I want. Sitting by the ocean places a purple gem of self-worth that holds its shine and doesn't lose its luster. Sleeping in on a Sunday morning and putting the chores aside improves my crown. Asking someone else to bake brownies for the bake sale secures that crown more securely on my head. I am a queen to my court of royalty.

Truth 44: Be a Little Messy

Living authentically allows the Universe to use you to help others move forward.

I was 23, a second-year elementary school teacher, and held great pride in the classroom that today would send any child with ADHD into a tailspin. The walls were cluttered with colorful posters, the decor was changed monthly according to the seasons, and everything was labeled. I welcomed my 20 first graders each morning with pride as those little ones were mine for the next 8 hours, and it was up to me to mother, nurture, and teach.

Ask any teacher to share with you particular students who have stood out in their teaching profession, and they will be quick to share their remembrances.

For the sake of anonymity, I will refer to one of my stand-out students as Holly. This little girl beat to her own drum. Her gait was light, a bit off, but somehow, she effortlessly floated through the classroom and shot baskets at gym class. The light brown curls that lined her forehead bounced untamed without much effort. She was always smiling, odd, and content with having a few close friends. She didn't seem to know any different. She was all of her in all of her being. She rolled with the punches and rarely was ruffled when a friend chose another over her. Her shoelaces were often untied, so I didn't even bother tying them for a fourth time each day. I think she might have been the one untying them for comfort. Her head was in the clouds, but her thoughts were magic. I know they were magic because I watched her draw.

Holly was a doodler. Her mom warned me at parent/teacher conferences that her daughter was obsessed with art and to be sure to put her back on track when she became lost in her drawings. Holly doodled on the corners of her morning work papers, desk, and backpack while waiting for the bus. It was the only time she was still. When she was drawing, she never sought out crayons or markers. She was content with a pencil. She never asked for a clean sheet of paper. She just drew on whatever she had available at the moment.

As her teacher, I spent lots of time redirecting her to ensure she took what she needed academically. At times, she was a frustrating student to teach, but overall, she was tolerable. She stood out amongst her peers as a one-of-a-kind type of kid. Quirky, adorable, and a complete mess.

She didn't fit the mold of a typical first-grader who was up on the most popular cartoon or superhero. She gravitated to the things that most kids knew nothing about. She would share her ideas with flair and have no reaction when her peers looked at her blankly. She didn't care because she had enough spice within her to keep her momentum for life up and lively.

One particular day, Holly was drawing faster than usual. She was immersed in her task as she bent over her desk, her tongue curled to her outer lip in concentration, without a hint of attachment to her surroundings. It was just her, a pencil, and a blank paper. I stood behind her without her knowing. I watched and tried to make sense of whatever story she was working hard to share. There were swirls, tiny people, stars, and raindrops. It was not the average first-grade drawing that resembled me and the student standing under a rainbow with a heart around our images. Holly's drawing was her soul throwing up all over a blank slate. This drawing would appear to the outsider as a chaotic mess, lacking structure. To Holly, this was her mind. I bent down and entered her circle only when I noticed her lean back and take in her masterpiece from a different vantage point.

I took the brief opportunity for her to share her drawing with me. I can't remember what she said or what it was about, but I do remember the shift in her persona when she became attached to what she had created. On paper, the drawing was messy. Scribbles, dark and light, weaving in and out of one another, trying to escape with nowhere to go. This was Holly. She was a mess. But that mess was filled with a fascinating beauty.

As a teenager, I would flip through the magazine "Sixteen" with envy. The sculpted bodies, airbrushed hair, and tiny waists taunted me. I wanted to be these girls. I tried to carry this image. I wanted to be perfect, just like them. I attempted to replicate the fashions using items from Walmart and Old Navy. Still, they never worked too well —the celebration in these types of magazines involved having it all together without one blemish to reveal. Nothing was messy in these magazines, and everything was perfect. However, it was only perfect because the imperfections were disguised through airbrush techniques and editing.

As a teen, it didn't take me long to recognize that this ideal was highly unattainable. But yet, like most teens, I still let the taunting get to me.

Many years later, it took a quirky six-year-old to teach me about the beauty of mess. Just one look at her, and her associated artwork changed me. She owned who she was and what she produced, which fascinated me. Not once did she do things for the approval of others. She did things according to what she knew she needed to for her soul self. Her mess, as interpreted by some, was instead a reflection of who she was at her core. And she was brave enough to live it without inhibition.

Hanging on my kitchen wall is a quote by one of my favorite authors, activists, and podcaster, "Be messy and complicated and afraid and show up anyway" (Glennon Doyle Melton). My kitchen wall holds this quote for my children, not for me to read. I hope it offers some courage for them to own who they are, screw up, and see it as something beautiful in the end. This quote evokes the same feeling I had when I first discovered Jackson Pollock's artwork. Colorful chaos, singing a symphony distinct to that particular canvas. We are our canvas.

I choose now to live this life a little bit messy. The energy it takes to quiet the distorted brilliance is too much work. Unleashing the power of disorder has the potential to lead to something you didn't know was there. I'm not suggesting we become complacent and give up on our goals and health. Instead, I feel a challenge to live life according to the philosophy of "I have no fucking clue what I'm doing, but I'm trusting the process along the way."

And the way we trust the process of this life, which we often call a mess, means that we must stay grounded in our true selves. What is that? What does the phrase "true self" mean? It means you challenge yourself not to be afraid to be like Holly. If you know you are different, you probably are. If you know there's something you are called to do, then you should do it. If you know you are living a lie, it's time to come clean. The true self will reveal itself to you in the loudest of whispers.

Let go of the reins and watch life deliver you a basket of treats at the most appropriate times. Living authentically allows the Universe to use you to help others move forward. Through this process, we allow others to be set free and learn that we can be our authentic selves, ultimately benefiting from it. Don't think for a second that the mistakes we make in life are just mistakes. They are beautiful messes disguised.

Truth 45: Protect Your Time

It should be intentional and soaked with purpose if I am to give my time to someone or something.

According to the most recent CDC statistics, a human's average life expectancy is 79.25 years. (October, 2024) Considering this statistic, I am more than halfway there, with a significant hiccup along the way. Years pass, Kids grow up, and the older we get, the more funerals we find ourselves attending for people who left imprints. The hardest are the ones where our hearts were imprinted more than our being.

Life is to be handled with care. It's tumultuous at times and seamless at others. In the end, it's short. So very short. When we are twenty, we feel invincible. In our thirties, we begin to thrive with our careers and still feel important. In our forties, we are confident and mostly secure in who we have become. We wonder how we've arrived at this point in our fifties so quickly, but we are hopeful that there is still much life to live. In our sixties, we understand what matters in life. We are grateful for good health in our seventies, but fully aware of the delicate balance we carry with each passing year, marked by the increasing candles on a birthday cake.

Something I learned through my sickness is that people do what they want to do. The ones I thought would be my biggest support throughout the long and lonely days were the ones who were the most distant. The ones I interacted with on a surface level came to be the ones whose hearts were the most generous and ran the deepest. These texts, interactions, or meals all shared one thing in common. Time. These individuals made time for me, and this equated to love.

And this simple lesson informed me how precious our time is. It should be intentional and soaked with purpose if I am to give my time to someone or something. Too many of us spread ourselves so thin that the time we give to things might as well be nothing, as we are barely present. Instead, we rush to get to the next thing. This is not living. This is slowly depleting yourself as your body isn't allowed to be present. It's rushed, hurried, and dismissed when all it wants to do is fully enjoy the moment. Cancer has taught me that time passes quickly, life is fleeting, and the time I spend during my quick-lived days should have a purpose. If the time spent with people or things does not support my overall well-being, I should evaluate my "why?" and choose to do things differently.

Years ago, a very dear man and mentor to Kyle and me during our early parenting years shared a phrase with me that I will forever return to. It's simple but powerful. "The most important gift you can give your children is your time." He was right. Reflect on your younger years and challenge yourself to bring forth memories where you felt emotionally secure. This security doesn't have to come from a parent's love. It can be anyone you were close to.

My dad was a hard worker. He strived to provide for us by ensuring we always had what we needed. He loved surprising us with big gifts at Christmas and always saving them for last to reveal as a surprise.

But the memory I attach to the most is the time spent throwing the softball after dinner. It was an act that didn't involve money or going

311

on a lavish vacation. It was just me, him, and a ball. On spring and summer nights, with a light breeze and the sun setting, I was the most important person to my dad at that moment. He would toss pop-up flyers and grounders, all the while giving pointers. I wanted to impress him because I wanted to make sure we could do this again. Sometimes, my sister would join in, and I welcomed that dynamic, but I preferred it just to be the two of us. I'm sure my dad was tired after a full day of work, but he put that aside and knew that the time spent with my sister and me was more important than sinking into the couch and decompressing.

Where we choose to spend our time is our decision. Often, we give up our time and commit to things without giving them a thought. We react without taking the time to consider how our decision to allocate resources will affect us. We are all allocated the same amount of time each day, and how we choose to divide it is entirely up to us. Begin challenging yourself to decide what best serves your energy.

I've learned that three categories in my life require the most time: family, friends, and career. When I separate this life trifecta, I can evaluate that family is the most important, but often the category given the least time. We must be proactive and mindful each day to pour the most into this category. Family is family. It doesn't change and, if ignored, only creates voids of space where emotional connection begins to disintegrate.

Time spent with friends is important because it's fulfilling and brings joy, but it's not as important as time with family.

Time spent working on our careers is necessary, but be mindful of how much time you allocate to this category. Some of us become so wrapped up in our profession that we become addicted to the financial and personal accolades, allowing these highs to overshadow where our time matters the most. Our families.

Before cancer, I worked a lot. Even while I was a stay-at-home mom, I found that I wasn't entirely present because I was planning and taking part in various side gigs. I'm not too hard on myself for this because our family did rely on this extra cash flow, and also because I found these gigs to be an outlet away from needy toddlers and crying babies.

As the kids became more independent, I briefly owned a yoga studio. I then single-handedly developed a very successful business that took over my life in such a way that it clouded my awareness of what mattered the most. My children. I was selfish with my work and believed I might lose it if I didn't give it all the time it deserved. However, I never once considered how my time spent on my business would take away from the time I could spend with my kids.

Don't get me wrong. I was still raising children, picking them up from school, and attending toddler story times at the library. I was physically present, but not mentally engaged. My brain held onto a daily post-it note list of things that needed to be done for my work to keep up with itself.

As much as I hate cancer, I will forever be grateful to it for the life lessons it has taught me. My business still runs, but at a minimal level. And I'm happy where it is because it no longer has a hold on me.

We are all allotted a certain amount of time in this world where we can become more of ourselves each day. We can either get stuck in the hamster wheel of moving through the motions or use our time to connect with others, learn, and explore. Most of us are unaware of the sacred minutes that float each day. This is normal as we become comfortable with our daily routines. Challenge yourself to be a bit retrospective on how you spend your time. Say no to the things that deplete you. Say yes to the things that grow and excite you. Make time for the ones you love. The family members who might rub you the wrong way. This is still time well spent. You will not regret the gestures in the end. Spend time alone and learn to be okay with it. When we are alone, mini-discoveries occur because others around us don't influence us.

This past year, I made it a goal to treat myself to a weekly date night. I am mostly successful if soccer practices and games don't interfere. I was uncomfortable amidst the older couples and bumble dates at the beginning of this commitment. Over time, I have come to embrace this time alone. I have a light pink Cosmo while watching NFL reruns and Little League Baseball Championships. The sweetness of these moments is for me and no one else. I have learned to be my own company. At times, friends have offered to join me. I don't take them up on it because my time is too precious. And it is especially precious when I'm giving it to myself.

Truth 46: *Stay Gold*

God sees our tarnish as His project to repair and protect.

As hard as I tried, I was never a reader. I collected the obligatory chapter books from the town library for the summer reading challenge, but usually got through about half of a Ramona Quimby book. I liked the feeling of carrying the treasures I borrowed from the library in the brown paper bag on loan for the summer. But the books sat next to my bed from June to late August. It wasn't until my eighth-grade English class that I discovered the profound impact a fictional story can have on my development. The Outsiders, written by S.E. Hinton, defied the script I was expected to follow in life. A set of misfit boys, thick as thieves, smarter than they gave themselves credit for, and lessons learned through hard choices. I resonated with them on some level, but a particular part of the story stood out to me.

Ponyboy, the main character, developed an appreciation for literature despite coming from a lower socioeconomic class. While hiding away with his trusted friend Johnny, he comes across a poem by Robert Frost. He reads it aloud to Johnny because he can't not. It's affected him on some soul level, and he wants to share it with someone.

Nothing Gold Can Stay

Nature's first green is gold,
Her hardest hue to hold.
Her early leaf's a flower;
But only so an hour.
Then leaf subsidies to leaf.
So Eden sank to grief,
So dawn goes down to day.
Nothing gold can stay.

Ultimately, the book encapsulated the idea that staying true to our identity is one of the most valuable aspects. Ponyboy was touched by this poem, not because of the flow of words or the introduction to great poetry, but because he felt himself through the words. He was a good, kind, honest, and lost boy trying to do the right thing. Without spoiling the story's outcome, the phrase "stay gold" carries a heavy weight that seeps deeply into the reader.

What does it mean to stay gold? I've thought about this a lot and wonder why this phrase resonates deeply. I've concluded that to "stay gold" means to embrace all of who you are in the most precious and beautiful ways. Seeing that gold takes millions of years to manifest, it's up to us to hold dear the golden parts of who we are and not take them for granted. Staying gold is a call to continue to be a good person and celebrate the gifts we are given. Especially the gifts we don't ask for.

To stay gold means recognizing the "why" behind the calling. When we see ourselves as separate from the usual metals of life, we make strides forward. Knowing that we are gold means knowing that we are good. Knowing that we are good means we have a positive impact on the world, whether we are aware of it or not. It takes an active mindset to settle into the knowing that we are valuable.

Many of us struggle to believe that we are valuable. I've struggled with this but discovered the secret to finding my worth. It's very simple: Tell yourself every day that you are worthy. You are not only deserving of good things; you are worthy of great things. Seeing yourself as gold is the first step, but polishing and embodying your worth takes years of work, daily work, and sometimes minutes.

In Scripture, gold is often described as precious and sacred. It's representative of the sun and understood as durable. I like to think that this is how Christ views us—polished, radiant, and beautiful in our way. It's hard to embody that we are loved and admired in such a way. Again, it falls back on our deep-seated wound of not feeling worthy. I'm challenging you and me to embrace the gold running through your veins. Scripture states, "All glorious is the princess in her chamber, with robes interwoven with gold" (Psalm 45:13). Melt into that word picture and embody for a moment that this is how we are called to view ourselves. Daily, your body takes care of you physically. Energetically, your body sends subtle alarms and intuitions throughout the day. Your life is yours; you have one, and it aches for you to admire its brilliance in the sun.

Sometimes, I think we get stuck in regrets about our past choices and don't consider that being gold is still available. We stay stuck, believing that being tarnished and scratched up is where we must live. We don't. We are children of God, and God is light. Therefore, we are light. And we are light underneath the luster of mistakes. A practice of discovering our worthiness is to begin forgiving ourselves and gently polishing the parts of us that are the hardest to look at.

Imagine a golden figurine tucked away in your grandmother's curio cabinet. Maybe it was a 50th wedding anniversary gift that was admired once but then found its place on a shelf among other figurines. However, once this gold piece is handled with care and polished, it exudes a radiance it was capable of underneath the layer of grime and dust. We are all gold, all good, and perfect beneath the thin layers of guilt and regret. God sees our tarnish as His project to repair and protect. Melt into the knowing that you deserve to feel valuable and of great worth. Staying gold means refining daily. Ask yourself if the choices you are making will make you shine brighter or dim your spirit. In time, you will notice that people are attracted to your gold. This is your energy. This is the vibration you are emitting. Ultimately, people respond to your energy more than to your actions.

Staying gold doesn't just happen. It's a constant reflection upon where we find ourselves in this world. The people we associate with, our connection to faith, and our willingness to do the work that comes with refining ourselves. In the end, the goal is that our gold will leave flakes of remembrance behind for our family and friends and be carried to the heavens just as Johnny had asked Ponyboy to do.

Truth 47: It's Okay to Outgrow

The unrest of staying with things that do not serve us should be enough to gently usher you forward.

Over the past few years of my adulthood, I have come to realize that very few people take the time to assess their growth. I get this. It's much easier to slide through the channels of life, as there is comfort in sameness and knowing what's coming next. Maybe I'm different in that I want to break through personal barriers to discover more of who I am and, more importantly, who I'm meant to be. Many of us get stuck in the mindset that relationships, jobs, and specific titles are permanent. They are not. They are only this way if we decide to make them this way. Often, we are so wrapped up in our life routine that ten years pass, and we find ourselves in the same headspace, a few pounds heavier, and with more wrinkles to show for it.

Since my diagnosis, I have embraced the inner awareness that I have a short time here to invest in those around me, but most importantly, myself. If we believe that we are all created with a purpose, why wouldn't we want to explore and strive to find that purpose with each passing day? This process doesn't have to be fast-moving; it's better if it's slow. Slow means asking yourself questions about why you feel a certain way. Slow means stopping to breathe. Slow means stepping onto the ledge to see what you could be, rather than where you think you should be. Slow thoughts are healing thoughts, and all are meant to foster a better relationship with yourself, which in turn serves you better in all other interactions we face.

For most of my life, I've stayed stuck out of fear of hurting another. I became used to living a half-fulfilling life to appease and please others. All the while depleting and ignoring what I could be used for. Making others happy was more important to me than making myself happy. To this day, I'm still learning and trying to figure out what happiness feels like. I've realized that happiness doesn't have to be big and grandiose. It can be sitting on my couch, the dog pushed up against my leg, willing me to pet her while I fold laundry. There is happiness in this moment because you choose to feel it.

One of the primary reasons people choose to turn the other cheek when it comes to fostering their well-being is because they feel attached to the things in life that have a hold on them. We can't grow if we choose to stay stuck, and we can't grow if we don't believe it's okay to outgrow. As I've already shared regarding the seasons of life, we need to continually challenge ourselves to view relationships in this way. I've become an expert at recognizing and sensing when a friendship is waning.

It's important to understand that often, this person did nothing wrong. Instead, I've done the work and no longer need them to the capacity that I once did. I offer this advice with a gentle and humble tone. When you slow down and dig into the shift that you already feel this friendship taking, you will be asked to either go with it or stay stuck in something that doesn't feel right. Eventually, if brave enough, you will move on because you won't have a choice not to. The unrest of staying with things that do not serve us should be enough to gently usher you forward.

Understand that others will notice this and may feel put off as you grow into your whole self. They will see a shift in your confidence and willingness to take risks, especially if that risk is stepping back from a friendship with them. There will be many times when you will feel a sense of isolation and loneliness. That's okay because it's here that you can practice self-discovery. It's like a small, green slate board we used in grammar school. Take the eraser, wipe away the dusty white chalk, and draw a new picture. When others respond with subtle, passive-aggressive attempts to interrupt your journey, respond in love and understand that this is their shit and not yours. Your self-growth and decision to move toward what fulfills you have nothing to do with how they knowingly or unknowingly react to you.

The process of outgrowing is a higher calling for many of us and is much easier said than done. But as we dip our toes into what it feels like, we will quickly discover that living here is much more fulfilling than living in sameness and predictability. Furthermore, if you don't move on from where you are, you do a disservice to those around you. You are keeping them stuck and comfortable. It's not our primary job to help others with their growth, but our responsibility is to allow them to discover their power by watching ours light up the sky.

I recently had a friend ask me if Kyle and I were divorced. She was timid when asking, feeling as though she had crossed some unspoken friendship line. I didn't blame her for asking, because Kyle and I weren't vocal about this decision. I immediately put her at ease with a smile and nod, saying, "It was so much better for our family." At that moment, I saw her admiration. No words, just a shift in how my story of bravery might resonate with her future tale of courage. People often watch and learn from how others navigate this world. Seeing that no one knows what we're doing, we take cues from those around us. It makes sense that we are inspired by motivational podcasts and books about others taking risks without knowing the outcomes. It's because we can't imagine doing those things ourselves. With this mindset, we become key players in assisting others through their self-development journey by challenging ourselves in ours.

Outgrowing relationships will cause some to talk about you behind your back. It's okay, they have work to do. People may employ subtle and passive-aggressive tactics to harm you. It's okay, they have work to do. They will be jealous of your risk-taking and unsure of how to handle your love and detachment simultaneously. They will build a wall of protection. That's okay, they have work to do.

Their work is not your work. Your work is your work, and the most important of all. I promise that the more you invest in the sculpture of who you are becoming, the more you feel at rest. Staying in what doesn't serve us feels uncomfortable. Growing out of something means that you are meant to grow into something. Why would we want to interrupt a process that wants nothing but to beautify itself?

I want my girls to grow up knowing that their mother is strong. As I currently navigate the teen years with my girls, I feel like I'm swimming upstream without a map to follow. I've learned it's best to stay in my lane, offer boundaries, offer connection, and say "I love you" whenever they leave the house. If I had chosen to stay in a loveless marriage, I believe they would see fear. If I had chosen to remain associated with particular friends, they would see submission. If I decided not to fight for my life, I believe they would not have me.

This process of outgrowing ripples extends to the ones we love the most, especially our children. Though my teens may not confess it now, they will someday reflect on the tough choices I made to better myself. I do not doubt that they will find themselves in similar situations, and it's my prayer, as their mom, that they see the beauty of what a larger pot can offer. We are all meant to bloom. And not bloom just once but over and over and over again. Do not limit what you know you could be because you are too afraid of how others might be made to feel. Instead, believe that your choice to grow taller will show them they have this same capacity. Your growth and outgrowing are unending, but the potential in the process is all that matters.

Truth 48: Stay in Your Power

When your power is practiced, it becomes refined over time, and through refinement, you discover things that have been hiding there all along.

Like most other Gen Xers, I was raised in a home where respect was first, followed by obedience, and compliance was expected. I agree with half of this parenting strategy as these principles are lacking today, but big aspects were also missing. We were taught to learn our lessons the hard way. Yet, there was no follow-up discussion on how the lesson affected us. We were taught that rules were there to keep us safe, but when we broke them and got caught, there was discipline without discussion. Our gifts weren't celebrated, and there wasn't much encouragement to explore how we could impact the world. Being "seen and not heard" seemed to be the theme of our upbringing, and we learned to deal with it. We had no other choice.

I was about sixteen or seventeen. The age when being around your parents felt suffocating for absolutely no reason at all. They talk, and you cringe. They suggest something, and you think they are crazy, but you take the advice without them knowing about it. You need them for food, clothes, and shelter to survive, so you deal with these aliens that you can't believe are the people you are stuck with.

Standing near our kitchen sink, my mom is next to me. She says something that upsets me or, more likely, something I disagree with her about. It's that time in my late teen development that I'm on the precipice of becoming someone with a voice. Until then, I tried not to cross my parents, challenge them, or call them out.

I stayed in my lane, did my best to follow the rules, and asked for forgiveness through prayer when I broke them. My mom threw down the dish towel on our kitchen counter, frustrated with whatever our little spat was about. I lashed out and stood my ground; words flew out of my mouth, and I didn't know where they came from. When I finished, we were both silent.

She looked at me and took a breath; she smiled, and everything in her changed. I didn't know what to expect for a moment and braced myself for a possible punishment. Instead, she cocked her head, locked eyes with me, and said, "Sarah, I'm proud of you! You said what you were feeling. Good for you!"

Whatever happened after that moment, I don't recall. However, I remember what I felt, and it was new. My stomach felt tingly, my chest more open, and my breathing deepened. Upon reflection, it was the first time in my life that I felt and discovered that I had a power that I was just being introduced to. I was surprised by how quickly this little fire rose to the surface and floated off my tongue like a match to a flame. Quick, immediate, hot, and impactful.

I tucked this feeling away and didn't practice using it for a long time. I always practiced it in my head, but when it came to disputes or arguments with friends, I followed my pattern of submission and let the other person have the right attitude. I knew my voice, but I didn't believe I had the right to feel what it desperately wanted to say.

After my illness, I learned that the more we quiet our internal power, the more we diminish the potential that is eagerly waiting to be discovered. This is why I felt so empowered when my mom affirmed my strength. My power was there; she felt it and acknowledged through her words that I was someone separate from her and was allowed to own my thoughts as my own. I started to explore my budding power in my early 40s by challenging others on why they held certain opinions. This might seem super simple, but to me, it was hard. I wasn't raised to think critically, disagree with others, or speak my mind. I found that, over time, this newly discovered superpower I had was kind of exciting. People taught me, and I taught them. We might disagree, but in the end, it was all okay.

When your power is practiced, over time, it becomes refined, and through this refinement, you uncover things that have been hidden all along. When these little discoveries of truth are brought to the surface, embrace them! Those discoveries are yours. They are to be held gently and protected. You don't need to share those discoveries with anyone. They won't care anyway. Trust me, I've tried. Instead, imagine that you are creating a sculpture of yourself with some of the strongest elements in the universe.

The tricky part about discovering your power is learning how to maintain it. It's easy to feel our power at certain times, particularly in how we respond to others when we disagree. It's easy to work on our power through self-talk when battling against the mind's lies. But it is a different calling to stay in the power of our entire being. I like to think of our inner power as a set of triplets. They are all genetically the same, but serve three distinct purposes. This trifecta represents our physical, mental, and spiritual power. When this beautiful summer storm of self-empowerment works together, we are one unstoppable force of intuition.

We are given one physical body. We are given the option to either care for it or allow its capabilities to deteriorate slowly. We are all familiar with the basics of maintaining our physical well-being. Still, we are also daily challenged with creature comforts, which include sweets, not going to the gym, or not challenging ourselves to give up our nicotine addiction.

We know how to feel better physically, but it's hard. We admire others who run with ease, their muscles sculpted, their gates perfect, while we sit in our cars at a red light, sipping our sugary, high-calorie drinks from Dunkin. *Good for them,* we say to ourselves. We know we should be doing something similar, but we'll set that thought aside for now, with the idea that we may start next week.

Step into a new mindset of understanding that your body wants you to feel good. It wants to be respected and cared for. It wants you to know that there is a better way to live where movement feels secure and less painful, clothes fit a bit looser, and sleep comes naturally. The cells within you make up your entire being. They are entrusted to you, and only you care for them. If you take care of them, they will take care of you.

Mental power comes in many forms and is the most complicated trifecta of strength. Your mental power is your ability to talk yourself off a ledge of untrue thoughts, stand firm in your belief system, or stay on a path you know you need to follow. It's practiced, it's hard, but it's so worth it in the end. I learned mental power at mile 19 of the marathons I ran in my twenties. The race day would arrive after months of training, icing, and tapering. You couldn't control the weather, so instead, you hoped for the best, and

327

if that 70-degree weather was replaced by wind and rain, that was what you had to deal with.

No marathoner backs out of a race because of the weather. There's too much invested at that point not to step on the chalk line. I found that, although every race had its personality, one thing was true for all of them. It came down to mile 19. My race was predicted up until that point. I knew my body well enough to know what would happen between miles one and nineteen. I knew when my calves would start to get sore and were on the verge of cramping. I knew what miles I would float through and where the annoying thoughts of self-doubt would try to taunt me.

However, for some reason, mile 19 was the one that attempted to alter the trajectory of the last 7 miles. Its job was either to break me or strengthen me. This is where I first learned of mental power. I now understand that mile 19 prepared me for the longest mile 19 of my life. July 15, 2022, I look up the long and steep hill of mile nineteen—the day of my Leukemia diagnosis. I'm grateful for mile 19.

Spiritual power is the quieter personality of the triplets, yet it holds the heaviest impact in shaping our character of strength. Though I was raised in a non-denominational Christian faith and recognize Christ as my Father, I don't expect everyone to feel or follow the same path. I have come to respect every religion and am fascinated by the ways others worship. I will respect the faith choices that work for individuals. Some might disagree with me, and that's okay, but I firmly believe that we should all connect with a higher power. I suggest this because we are not enough when asked to rely solely on physical and mental strength. Given that our bodies are highly energetic, it makes sense to support ourselves with spiritual guidance when our psychological and physical aspects tire.

Next to my bed in my hospital room sat devotionals and my bible. Sometimes I didn't want to look at them because I was mad at God for causing this shit storm in my body. Of course, this is not the case, but a lie I would occasionally return to. At other times, I would open the pages and cry tears of relief when I heard His voice through the words of Scripture that carried me. When we choose not to explore our spiritual potential, we limit the full power we could have.

Physical, mental, and spiritual powers want to be your guides and stand alongside you in every facet of your life. Daily challenge yourself to stay in all three of your superpowers. This takes time, diligence, bravery, tenacity, and patience as you learn what is right for you and what is not. In the end, the power of you will float you to the top of the steepest peaks of your mile 19s.

Truth 49: Don't Wait

When we don't honor what we already know, we suffocate what we know we could be.

I close this book with what I find to be the most essential truth to live by. It took me 49 days of hospital isolation and a potential death sentence for me to reflect upon all the waiting I had done over the years. After multiple restoration steps, I waited for my marriage to feel a spark of life again. I chose to bypass bravery and sit in sadness. I decided to stay in the firing squad of tasks and say yes to everything thrown my way. I decided to wait, knowing there was something better for me than the life I was living. I chose to stay rather than move. And I stayed because fears kept me bound.

When we don't honor what we already know, we suffocate what we know we could be. Again, we are doing a disservice to the gift of life we have been granted. Our bodies can only withstand so much neglect at the cellular level. It knows its worth and importance and, in time, will tell you that you have failed it.

Whether we acknowledge it or not, we must begin to understand that we are all here for a purpose. These purposes can start small, but when believed in and nurtured, they can grow into something greater than you ever expected. Every day, there are whispers inside of you guiding you. And we are very good at ignoring the ones that might be hard to hear. It's like someone telling you what a good musician or athlete you are, but you can't embrace it because you are the one in the way, unable to believe it. And it's the quietest whispers that

330

produce the greatest reward. Deep in the caverns of your heart are all the truths just waiting to be seen.

We all know how quickly this life passes. It takes just one look at a niece or nephew suddenly graduating from college to reflect on where 23 years have gone. And as much as I dislike using the word "shame," I think it applies well to the following sentence. Wouldn't it be a shame to live this life, year after year, snuffing out the whispers of truth that want to make you into the best version of yourself? This is not something to ignore and say you will get to later. Later can be too late. This life is so short. It is so brief, and we intuitively know that anything can change instantly. But this is a fleeting thought for most. Unfortunately, it is not a fleeting thought for others like me who have come so close to death; it feels blinding. You have to trust something bigger than you. And that something is already inside of you.

During my sickness, I created a short list of things I commit to doing before I die. So far, I've crossed off one. Seeing Bruce Springsteen live this past summer, with sand between my toes and the Jersey shore waves crashing close by. It was a clear night that seemed too perfect to be real. Bruce ends the night with "Jersey Girl," a song that carries a story I believe will sync up perfectly with my life once love finds me again.

Another item on my bucket list is to fly in a hot air balloon. I want to feel the ground beneath me as I step into the basket, ready to take flight. I want to feel connected to who I once was—the girl scared to take flight. I want to feel the fire and heat above me, soft sounds of power preparing me for my flight. I want my body to feel the parallel connection to the inner fire that has been found within me over the past two years. I want to fly high and watch the things below me become smaller and smaller the farther I go up. All these things remain the same. I do not. I'm moving. The heat, the height, and the power of this beautiful balloon hold the entirety of me. I will trust this vessel to carry me safely, and I look down upon the life I once lived and believe that I can keep soaring as long as I trust the process.

Step into the power of you. Don't wait for the opportunities to come to you. Lean on the doors, seek what inspires you, and trust the process. You don't need a blueprint. You need your intuition. And the most beautiful thing about intuition is that when we practice it, we refine it and give it wings to take us places. Quiet your heart and listen for the answers. And it's here that you discover the most beautiful being on the planet.

You.

She Said Yes

She walked to the edge, her gaze stretching as far as the horizon. Her eyes squinted, not against the sun, but in an inherent human quest to see beyond the visible—a natural inclination she'd often observed in others, now claiming her. She wasn't searching for anything specific, nor did she have a clear hope; she knew she was finally home.

Standing there, barefoot, her toes burrowed into the damp earth, finding a security she desperately craved. Her life had been a series of unexpected potholes, sharp twists, and abrupt turns, marked by a lack of predictability.

She'd managed it all by numbing, by succumbing, carrying a sting no bandage could ever truly heal.

But here, her shoulders relaxed, and she drew a deep breath, whispering, "Yes." If this journey meant walking alone, she was content, for it was in solitude that she found her deepest confidence and made her most beautiful discoveries.

Self-Reflective Study Guide

This study guide invites you to explore the book's profound truths and embark on a journey of self-discovery. By engaging in writing, contemplation, or group discussion, you'll uncover insights into your actions, acknowledge your successes, and cultivate remarkable personal growth.

Truth 1:
You are the Most Important Person

1. On a scale of 1 to 10, with 10 representing the maximum, how much of your time do you feel you're currently giving to those around you or to commitments you feel obligated to fulfill?

2. Identify five activities or commitments you don't enjoy or aren't genuinely invested in. Imagine omitting two or three of these from your life. How would this shift impact your daily routines, particularly on an emotional level?

3. Take a moment to reflect: Are you consistently putting your own needs aside to appease or please others? If you find yourself struggling to value yourself first, delve into the deeper roots of this pattern.

Truth 2:
Don't Hide Your Pain

1. When you reflect on the challenging situations you've overcome, how would you describe your approach to their emotional effects at the time and in the aftermath?

2. For those moments of heartache, loss, disappointment, grief, or fear that you don't openly share with loved ones, what underlying fears prevent you? How do you anticipate your emotions or body might respond if you were to share?

3. Are there any emotional experiences or traumas you've consciously kept hidden? Consider if you're prepared to embark on a journey of self-discovery and healing, even if it's just through gentle, initial steps, to confront these feelings.

Truth 3:
Good is Good Enough

1. Consider if you tend to be a people pleaser. If this resonates, what kind of affirmation or emotional high do you experience when you put others' desires before your own?

2. Many describe themselves as Type A or perfectionists. Do you fit this description? If so, have you considered whether your upbringing shaped this tendency?

3. Imagine integrating the idea that "Good is Good Enough" into your life. In what ways could this perspective alter your daily patterns?

Truth 4:
Change It

1. Allow your immediate thoughts and feelings to guide you: what is one significant thing you would like to alter about your life?

2. Consider the most recent significant change you implemented in your life. How has that shift contributed positively to where you are today?

3. If you find yourself in a challenging situation, like an unhealthy relationship, an unfulfilling job, or an unhealthy lifestyle, what barriers are holding you back from initiating a transformation?

Truth 5:
The Valleys of Vulnerability

1. Based on this chapter, how would you define vulnerability to someone else?

2. When engaging in conversations, do you generally lean towards being vulnerable or transparent? And how do people typically respond to this open way of communicating with you?

3. If vulnerability isn't a practice you engage in, delve into the reasons why. Could it be linked to a perceived uncertainty or risk in how others might react to your deeper openness?

Truth 6:
Pain is Pain

1. Reflect on the most profound emotional pain you've experienced. How would you describe it?

2. How did your physical body respond to this intense emotional pain? Thinking about our nervous system's stress responses, did you tend to "fight," "flee," or "freeze" in the face of it?

3. Do you ever feel that others are dealing with "greater" pain than your own? If so, consider the reasons behind this perception, and then explore the complexities of your emotional struggles.

Truth 7:
Stop Chasing

1. Are you a "grass is greener" person? If so, where has this process of thinking benefited or hurt you in the past?

2. Take a moment for an honest self-assessment: What current pursuit is demanding an excessive amount of your time?

3. Reflect on the significance of seeking approval from others in your life. Does the idea of more money equate to true happiness for you? Is acknowledgment from colleagues a primary driver in your career? Consider the ways you might be striving for external validation, and then envision how your life might shift if you allowed opportunities to present themselves naturally.

Truth 8:
Nothing's "A Shame"

1. Based on your understanding, how would you explain the word "shame" to a close friend?

2. Allowing your first thought to emerge, what is the single thing you feel the most shame about, and what do you believe is its root cause?

3. Reflecting on your formative years, did shame become a concept you recognized and understood? Can you identify specific individuals who may have contributed to a sense of shame in your life?

Truth 9:
Dauntless

1. Reflect on the phrase "all things work together for those who are brave." What personal meaning does it hold for you?

2. Recall someone you know who made a difficult, brave choice. What positive results came from their courage?

3. Do you trust what might happen if you make the brave choice you know you need to make? How could this choice make your life more beautiful?

Truth 10:
Break the Cycle 2

1. Looking back at your upbringing, what unhealthy cycles had an impact on you?

2. How do those past cycles continue to impact your adjustment and responses in your present life?

3. Are there any unhealthy patterns you're aware of that you need to break? If so, what's preventing you from making that change?

Truth 11:
Say No

1. Do you often struggle to decline requests, commitments you lack interest in, or other situations that leave you feeling resentful?

2. When you say no to a person or a commitment, what emotional reactions do you notice within yourself?

3. Commit to saying 'no' to at least one thing in the coming weeks. Play out the conversation in your mind and consider the various ways people might react.

Truth 12:
Fear Has No Power

1. Consider the boundaries and limitations fear imposes on your life. Do you believe that if practiced, you can have power over your fears?

2. Identify your biggest fear related to change or your current life situation. Are you willing to take a baby step into change and challenge the fear?

3. Imagine speaking truth to this fear: what message would you deliver?

Truth 13:
Your Circumstances Do Not Define You

1. What present or past situation in your life brings about feelings of shame?

2. Consider how much mental energy this situation drains, diverting you from experiences that bring you happiness. How might your life transform if you diminished its hold?

3. Are you willing to embrace your mistakes, offer yourself forgiveness, and see them as stepping stones to greater understanding?

Truth 14:
If You Feel It, Do It

1. Reflect on a time when you felt the most joyful. Pinpoint the activities and passions that fueled that happiness, and consider how it would feel to revisit some of them.

2. What does your inner wisdom tell you to pursue when you allow yourself to be still?

3. What is holding you back from fully embracing your inner power and moving forward with what you want and need?

Truth 15:
Cry, Punch, or Throw Shit

1. Do you find the label for this truth unsettling? If so, where does that feeling originate?

2. What's your usual approach when you feel anger surfacing? Do you lean into it or push it away? Does anger have a hold on you, or do you feel as though you can navigate through it?

3. Visualize the release of this anger: Does it involve an honest conversation, a powerful physical release, or something else?

Truth 16:
Detach

1. What situation is your body urging you to release? Listen for an intuitive, not mental, response.

2. What's been the obstacle to taking that crucial first step towards detachment?

3. Name someone you admire who excels at setting boundaries. How do their actions and way of living demonstrate this?

Truth 17:
Strong Is a Choice

1. What are your thoughts on the statement, "Strength is a choice?" Do you see yourself as a strong person when facing life's difficult challenges or unexpected turns?

2. Do you feel that you rely too heavily on others during personal trials? When others offer advice, does it truly influence the way you respond and react to your situation?

3. Can you identify an area in your life where you might begin to choose strength over fear, even in small ways? What might that look like in your actions, and how do you imagine that choice would feel in your body?

Truth 18:
Listen

1. In conversation, do you often find yourself thinking about what you're going to say next while the other person is still speaking?

2. How would you describe the concept of "listening through vibrational exchange?" If that phrase feels unclear, consider this: how does another person's emotional state affect the way you listen and respond during a conversation?

3. Have you taken the time to truly listen to your inner voice or sense of inner knowing? Is there a message within you that you've been ignoring or hesitant to respond to?

Truth 19:
Be Conscious, Not Careless

1. Have you ever noticed that you rarely question your patterns or the relationships that surround you? I wonder if, in some way, this might come from a quiet reluctance-or even a forgotten curiosity—about what else life might have to offer.

2. What does it mean to live in your power, in a way that honors the truth of who you uniquely are?

3. Do you truly believe you are worthy of all the good things life has to offer? If your answer is yes, take a moment to explore why—what within you affirms that sense of worthiness? If your answer is no, gently ask yourself: Where might that feeling of unworthiness come from? Can you approach it with curiosity rather than judgment?

Truth 20:
Accept It

1. Regarding your past or present, what are some of the most challenging things you're struggling to embrace or come to terms with fully?

2. What are some of the aspects of who you are that you're struggling to come to terms with?

3. Close your eyes and picture it: What would it feel like to live as a version of yourself that fully accepts every facet of who you are?

Truth 21:
Just Love

1. As you reflect on Paul's words in 1 Corinthians 13:13, 'So now faith, hope, and love abide, these three; but the greatest of these is love,' what thoughts arise for you regarding why he might consider love to be the 'greatest'? Perhaps challenge yourself to explore what makes love distinct from hope or faith.

2. What does loving yourself truly mean to you? Beyond the instant gratification of a new purchase or the momentary relief of a Friday night massage, how are you actively cultivating this love in more profound ways? And, looking back, what aspects of yourself are you now learning to embrace that were once incredibly difficult to accept?

3. As you look inward, is there one person in your life to whom extending love feels particularly challenging? If you were to gently begin offering that grace, even just dipping a toe in, what might that look and feel like for you and for them?

Truth 22:
Energy is Honest

1. As you look back, can you recall an instance where you chose not to honor the quiet wisdom of your intuition? How did that decision resonate within you, and what did you learn from the way things unfolded afterwards?

2. Do you have a difficult time being still with yourself, in silence, with no noise or people, just you? If so, what thoughts are getting in the way? Do you have specific reasons related to emotional unrest?

3. As you consider the phrase, "Energy is Honest," what initial thoughts or feelings come to mind? How do you interpret what that title conveys about the nature of energy in our lives or interactions?

Truth 23:
Be a Truth Teller

1. As you tune into your own experience, how does stress manifest physically in your body? What are the common catalysts for these physical reactions? You may even begin to explore the idea of letting go of one specific stressor that weighs on you.

2. Reflecting on the sentiment, "Others' reactions to your honesty are a direct reflection of them, not you," what personal meaning do you draw from it? How might this perspective shift how you view complicated interactions?

3. As you consider fully living as your truth-telling self, what aspects of that journey do you anticipate might be challenging, and why? And yet, what positive outcomes might you also envision emerging from such an authentic way of being?

Truth 24:
Don't Get Stuck

1. Why do you think our brains sometimes seem to linger more on negative memories than on positive ones? When you bring both types of experiences to mind, which kind do you find yourself able to recall in richer, more vivid detail?

2. It can be not easy, but perhaps you might reflect on how you could begin to reframe a challenging thought, guiding it towards a more positive perspective. What possibilities emerge when you consider such a shift?

3. Thinking about your personal growth, what three affirmations resonate deeply with you that you could display on your bathroom mirror each morning? What specific words would help you cultivate a more positive mindset and support your journey of self-improvement?

Truth 25:
Manifest That Shit

1. When you consider faith alongside manifestation, what correlation or interplay do you believe exists? What are your thoughts on how these two ideas might be intertwined in the process of bringing things into being?

2. As you look ahead, what three things, actions, or heartfelt wishes would you genuinely love to bring into reality? More importantly, deep within yourself, do you sense that you possess the power to manifest them?

3. When you reflect on how intuition operates, do you sense a profound connection between it and the process of manifestation? How might that inner knowing serve as a direct link, guiding you towards the very things you hope to bring into your life?

Truth 26:
Ask for Help

1. Is it challenging for you to ask for help? If so, what might be the underlying reasons? Could pride or other personal factors be influencing this reluctance?

2. How do you respond when others ask you for help? Do you feel resentful, or are you willing to overextend yourself, even if it means neglecting your own needs?

3. If you're always the one offering help, how might it feel to say no occasionally? How could your life shift if you started setting that boundary, even just occasionally?

Truth 27:
Do The Scary

1. Take a moment to notice the first thing that comes to mind. What is something you want to do, but find yourself holding back from due to fear or self-doubt?

2. Take a moment to reflect on Robert Frost's words: 'Two roads diverged in a wood, and I–I took the one less traveled by, And that has made all the difference.' On a personal level, what does this quote mean to you? How might it relate to the choices you've made in your own life?

3. 'Life will test you, but it will always catch you.' Do you find truth in this statement? Why or why not? And if you're unsure, what might be standing in the way of fully believing it?

Truth 28:
What Lights You Up?

1. Think back to a time in your life when you felt happy. What were the activities, not the people, that brought you joy and sparked excitement in you?

2. What are three hobbies you'd like to revisit or new ones you'd like to explore? Which one sparks the most curiosity for you, and what steps could you take to begin pursuing it?

3. What's holding you back from reigniting a passion you've drifted from or starting one you're interested in? If time feels like a barrier, what might you be able to let go of to create more space for yourself?

Truth 29:
Shit Happens, But It's All Redeemed

1. What difficult situation are you currently facing? Do you believe this challenging moment will eventually pass, and could it hold a hidden blessing or valuable lesson in the process?

2. When faced with a challenge, do you tend to lean toward a positive or negative perspective? Take a moment to be honest with yourself about this.

3. If a close friend were to ask you how you're *really* doing, could you answer honestly? What would that response sound like?

Truth 30:
Forgive

1. What might it mean to do a disservice to yourself by withholding forgiveness, and how could this choice affect your healing and peace?

2. Think of one person you find it hard to imagine ever forgiving. Now, take a moment to close your eyes and picture yourself approaching them. You don't need to act on this – it's simply a way to start the inner process of forgiveness, even if you're not ready to fully let go. And that's perfectly okay.

3. How does this verse resonate with you? 'Lord, how many times should I forgive someone who sins against me? Up to seven times?' Jesus replied, 'I tell you, not seven times, but seventy-seven times.' (Matthew 18:21-35) How do these words challenge your understanding of forgiveness, and what might they reveal about your capacity to forgive?

Truth 31:
Grieve Hard

1. What is the deepest grief you've had to face? Can you allow yourself to feel it fully in this moment? Whether it's through tears, anger, or simply curling up in silence, it's okay. Healing begins when we allow ourselves to feel honestly.

2. What does it mean to honor someone you've lost by allowing yourself to grieve deeply, embracing whatever form that grief takes? How might fully feeling this loss be a way of honoring their memory and your healing process?

3. When it comes to the three stress responses—fight, flight, or freeze—which one does your body naturally lean towards? This isn't something you can control, but simply an awareness of how your inner wiring responds to stress.

Truth 32:
Four Friends

1. The phrase 'stay selfish for yourself' can carry a challenging ring. But what does it signify, and how does it resonate with you?

2. As we journey through life, the people who walk beside us often settle into distinct roles. What is the value of keeping your circle small, and do you feel as though yours is too large right now?

3. Consider your foundational friend: who is that steady presence, and what enduring impact have they had on the very bedrock of your life? Then there's the realist friend, the one who isn't afraid to challenge your views—how have they pushed you to adjust your perspective, truly becoming a teacher in your life? Who is your space-holder friend, that rare soul with whom you feel an unshakeable sense of safety, allowing you to be truly vulnerable? And what about seasonal friends? Who fills that role for you now, and who has in the past? Is there inherent value in these transient connections, and if so, what is it?

Truth 33:
It's Your Story

1. As we reflect on our journeys, we each carry a unique "story." Consider, then: are there parts of your story that you're apprehensive about sharing with others? And if so, can you pinpoint why that is?

2. What does it mean to embrace a life of transparency?

3. Explore how sharing your difficult life stories can be a source of healing and growth, not only for yourself but for those who bear witness to your journey.

Truth 34:
Discipline Delivers

1. Do you perceive yourself as someone who embodies discipline? As you reflect, notice the specific areas of your life where this quality, or perhaps its absence, becomes most apparent.

2. Think about a goal you either have or have been considering. Describe it briefly. Then, reflect on the specific ways daily discipline would manifest in your actions, habits, and choices to help you bring this goal to fruition.

3. Have you identified your innate gift, your life's calling, or what you are uniquely positioned to share with the world? If these concepts still feel undefined, pause and reflect on what the Universe is inviting you to step into.

Truth 35:
Broken is Beautiful

1. Who are the people that come to mind when you think about how they made you feel both positive and negative? How did their impact help to construct your character?

2. Reflect on the concept of translating 'hard to beautiful.' How can you shift your perspective and actively create beauty, meaning, or wisdom from challenging circumstances?

3. Are you willing to befriend the aspects of yourself you've felt shame about? Can you allow these once-hidden parts to transform and become a beautiful, authentic extension of who you are?

Truth 36:
Quit Judging

1. How quickly do you find yourself falling into patterns of judgment toward yourself and others?

2. Could your critiques of others stem from something you're avoiding within yourself? If so, be curious about what that is.

3. Do you find yourself heavily influenced by the judgments of others? Reflect on the concept that "like energy attracts like energy" in this context. What practical strategies can you implement to avoid becoming entangled in this cycle?

Truth 37:
Hurdles

1. Take a moment to identify one thing that feels overwhelming to you right now. This might be a looming project deadline, planning a significant event like a wedding, or navigating a challenging life transition such as a divorce or illness. As you consider this, reflect on your current headspace regarding the situation. Are you finding yourself in a state of avoidance, or are you willing to start setting mini goals to navigate it?

2. As you navigate your current challenge, take a moment to imagine: What would it feel like to reach the other end of this particular hardship?

3. Who are the individuals in your life whom you can lean on for emotional support?

Truth 38:
Guilt Will Destroy You

1. As you reflect on your journey, ask yourself: Is there an experience or action from your past that still causes you immense guilt?

2. To what extent does this guilt influence your life? Does it linger in the shadows of your thoughts, a topic you sidestep but frequently revisit internally?

3. Are you prepared to embark on the process of self-forgiveness, and if so, do you genuinely believe in your capacity to embrace it?

Truth 39:
People Will Hurt You, Get Used to It

1. Take a moment to reflect on Maya Angelou's insight: "When people show you who they are, believe them the first time." How does this quote resonate with specific scenarios or relationships you've experienced in your own life?

2. To what extent do the opinions of others affect you, and how much emotional energy do you find yourself dedicating to them?

3. How do you feel about the idea of sending love to someone who has hurt or wronged you? If this feels difficult, consider exploring the reasons why. Be curious about the potential outcome if you were to **genuinely** practice this way of living.

Truth 40:
Protect and Celebrate Your Gift

1. What is unique about you? What special quality or skill do you possess that is worth acknowledging and celebrating? It could be a musical talent, a form of artistic expression, a physical prowess, or an exceptional ability to forge connections with others. Identify this distinct part of your being.

2. Considering this unique gift or talent you've identified, have you limited or held back this inherent strength? If so, reflect on why that might be.

3. Consider someone you know who possesses a unique gift and appears to be using it to its fullest potential. How does their life serve as a reflection of the richness and fulfillment that comes from embracing and expressing that gift?

Truth 41:
Extend Grace

1. The book of Hebrews 4:16 reminds us: "Let us then with confidence draw near to the throne of grace, that we may receive mercy and find grace to help in time of need." As you reflect, how do you personally interpret and apply this verse to assure yourself that you are indeed deserving of grace, regardless of the mistakes you've made, whether recent or long past?

2. Take a moment to imagine: What would it feel like to practice extending grace to someone who has hurt or wronged you?

3. Reflect on the link between self-forgiveness and grace as it manifests in your own life.

Truth 42:
Death Does Not Hold You

1. If you've experienced deep grief, reflect on how you've navigated its intensity. Have you allowed yourself to sit in the pain fully, or have you avoided its heavy sting, perhaps out of fear of what might surface?

2. In what ways does embracing deep grief contribute to the journey of healing?

3. If your natural inclination is to hide your pain, what are some small, curious steps you can take to begin gently exploring it? And if you're not ready to take those steps right now, that's perfectly okay.

Truth 43:
Validation is Overrated

1. If this truth resonates, consider if your actions, or perhaps even a tendency towards over-scheduling, are driven by a quest for such validations.

2. If so, can this pursuit of external validation secretly foster resentment toward the very choices or actions that produce that validation?

3. What does it mean for you to live primarily from your heart, rather than solely from your head?

Truth 44:
Be a Little Messy

1. Consider Glennon Doyle's statement: "Be messy and complicated and afraid and show up anyway." What personal significance does this quote hold for you, and how does its message speak to your journey?

2. What if you were to step away from the internal script of how things *should* be and instead challenge the Universe or a higher power to direct your path?

3. Reflect on your journey: How has a past "mess" in your life been redeemed as something beautiful, even in the smallest of ways?

Truth 45:
Protect Your Time

1. What does this statement mean to you, and how do you resonate with it in your own life? "People do what they want to do."

2. On a piece of paper, draw a circle or a pie chart. Divide it into three sections representing Family, Friends, and Career. Based on your current time allocation, shade or proportion each section. Are you okay with how you're spending your time in each portion?

3. How comfortable are you with being alone, with no one else around? If you find these situations uncomfortable, explore the root of this feeling. What thoughts or emotions arise when you are alone?

Truth 46:
Stay Gold

1. Reflect on how the phrase "Stay Gold" resonates with you. If you are familiar with *The Outsiders*, consider why S.E. Hinton's phrase may have had a profound impact on the main character.

2. Reflect on your belief in being a child of God. How does the idea that He views you as a precious metal, worthy of protection and unconditional love (like a father loves a child), resonate with you?.

3. Considering this truth, what aspects of your life do you feel called to refine?

Truth 47:
It's Okay to Outgrow

1. What does it mean to have "done the work" as it applies to the slowing down or soft ending of friendships?

2. When people react, it is more often about "their shit, not yours." Can you think of a current or past scenario with a relationship where this idea might be applicable?

3. How does staying put, rather than embracing new opportunities, prevent you from helping others?

Truth 48:
Stay in Your Power

1. Define "staying in your power" concerning making authentic choices, forming congruent relationships, and consciously navigating energetic shifts.

2. Which of your body's three superpowers—physical, mental, or spiritual—do you rely on most confidently?

3. Do you believe you possess personal power? Why or why not?

Truth 49:
Don't Wait

1. Contemplate this statement: "When we don't honor what we already know, we suffocate what we know we could be." What does this mean to you? What are the first thoughts that come to mind when contemplating?

2. Right now, what is your intuition guiding you to do?

3. When and how will you begin? Finally, are you ready to trust the abundance awaiting you?

Fight Song
Rachel Platten, 2015

Like a small boat on the ocean
Sending big waves into motion
Like how a single word
Can make a heart open
I might only have one match
But I can make an explosion

And all those things I didn't say
Were wrecking balls inside my brain
I will scream them loud tonight
Can you hear my voice this time?

This is my fight song
Take back my life song
Prove I'm alright song
My power's turned on
Starting right now, I'll be strong

I'll play my fight song
And I don't care if nobody else believes
'Cause I've still got a lot of fight left in me

Losing friends and I'm chasing sleep
Everybody's worried 'bout me
In too deep, say I'm in too deep
And it's been two years, I miss my home
But there's a fire burning in my bones
Still believe, yeah, I still believe

And all those things I didn't say
Wrecking balls inside my brain I
will scream 'em loud tonight
Can you hear my voice this time?

This is my fight song
Take back my life song
Prove I'm alright song
My power's turned on
Starting right now, I'll be strong
I'll play my fight song
And I don't care if nobody else believes
'Cause I've still got a lot of fight left in me

A lot of fight left in me

Like a small boat on the ocean
Sending big waves into motion
Like how a single word
Can make a heart open
I might only have one match
But I can make an explosion

This is my fight song
Take back my life song
Prove I'm alright song
My power's turned on
Starting right now, I'll be strong
I'll play my fight song
And I don't care if nobody else believes
'Cause I've still got a lot of fight left in me

No, I've still got a lot of fight left in me

Resources

American Cancer Society. (n.d.). *Cancer.org*. Retrieved from https://www.cancer.org/

Callan D. Costa Foundation. (n.d.). *Callan D. Costa Foundation*. Facebook. Retrieved from https://www.facebook.com/cdcfoundation0615/

CancerCare. (n.d.). *CancerCare*. Retrieved from https://www.cancercare.org/

Cancer Support Community. (n.d.). *Cancer Support Community*. Retrieved from https://www.cancersupportcommunity.org/

Childhood Leukemia Foundation. (n.d.). *Childhood Leukemia Foundation*. Retrieved from https://www.clf4kids.org/

Cornwall, D. J. (2014). *Things I wish I'd known: Cancer caregivers speak out*. American Cancer Society.

Daniel P. Ryan Foundation. (n.d.). *The Daniel P. Ryan Foundation*. Retrieved from https://dprf.org/

Ekakitie, M. T., & Johnson, C. B. (2020). *Beyond the diagnosis: Surviving and thriving with multiple myeloma and breast cancer*. Independently published.

Green, T., & Dachinger, D. (2020). *Live calm with cancer (and beyond): A patient & caregiver guide to finding more ease through the power of mindfulness*. Green & Dachinger.

Giusti, K. (2021). *Fatal to fearless: 12 steps to beating cancer in a broken medical system*. Hachette Go.

Hackensack Meridian Health. (n.d.). *Cancer navigator program at John Theurer Cancer Center in NJ: Your cancer journey advocate*.

Retrieved from https://www.hackensackmeridianhealth.org/en/ services/cancer-care/nurse-navigators

Hackensack Meridian Health. (n.d.). *Cancer support services in New Jersey | John Theurer Cancer Center | Hackensack Meridian Health*. Retrieved from https://www.hackensackmeridianhealth.org/ en/services/cancer-care/cancer-support-services

Hackensack Meridian Health. (n.d.). *Find support groups near you*. Retrieved from https://www.hackensackmeridianhealth.org/en/ about-us/support-groups

Hackensack Meridian Health. (n.d.). *Leukemia treatment in NJ | Hackensack Meridian John Theurer Cancer Center*. Retrieved from https://www.hackensackmeridianhealth.org/en/services/cancer-care/ leukemia

Joe's House. (n.d.). *Joe's House*. Retrieved from https:// www.joeshouse.org/

Kalanithi, P. (2016). *When breath becomes air*. Random House.

Leukemia Research Foundation. (n.d.). *Leukemia Research Foundation*. Retrieved from https://leukemiarf.org/

The Leukemia & Lymphoma Society. (n.d.). *Light The Night*. Retrieved from https://www.lightthenight.org/

The Leukemia & Lymphoma Society. (n.d.). *The Leukemia & Lymphoma Society*. Retrieved from https://www.lls.org/

The Leukemia & Lymphoma Society. (n.d.). *Support resources*. Retrieved from https://www.lls.org/support-resources

Lymphoma Research Foundation. (n.d.). *Ticketed events*. Retrieved from https://lymphoma.org/waystohelp/ticketedevents/

Mukherjee, S. (2010). *The emperor of all maladies: A biography of cancer*. Scribner.

OncoLink. (n.d.). *OncoLink*. Abramson Cancer Center of the University of Pennsylvania. Retrieved from https://www.oncolink.org/

Ronald McDonald House Charities. (n.d.). *Ronald McDonald House Charities*. Retrieved from https://www.rmhc.org/

Smelcer, J. E. (2015). *Running from the reaper: Poems from an impatient cancer survivor*. University of Alaska Press.

St. Jude Children's Research Hospital. (n.d.). *St. Jude Children's Research Hospital*. Retrieved from https://www.stjude.org/

9 798986 023571